Table Of Contents

History and Philosophy of Ayurveda 3
Ayurveda for Beginners: Enhancing Your Health and Beauty
Naturally 3
Determining Your Dominant Dosha 3
Benets of Ayurveda for Health and Beauty 3
Principles of Ayurveda 3
Benets of Ayurveda for Health and Beauty 3
Vata Dosha: Characteristics and Imbalances 3
Ayurveda for Beginners: Enhancing Your Health and Beauty
Naturally 3
Pitta Dosha: Characteristics and Imbalances 3
Benets of Ayurveda for Health and Beauty 3
Ayurveda for Beginners: Enhancing Your Health and Beauty
Naturally 3
Online Resources for Ayurvedic Information 3
Ayurvedic Practitioners and Retreats 3
Ayurveda and Certication Programs 3
Ayurveda for Beginners: Enhancing Your Health and Beauty
Naturally 3
Continuing Your Ayurvedic Journey 3
Ayurveda for Beginners: Enhancing Your Health and Beauty
Naturally 3
Recap of Ayurvedic Principles and Practices 3
Embracing Ayurveda for Enhanced Health and Beauty 3
Your Ayurvedic Journey Begins Now! 3
Ayurveda for Beginners: Enhancing Your Health and Beauty
Naturally 3
Ayurveda for Beginners: Enhancing Your Health and Beauty
Naturally 3
Ayurveda for Beginners: Enhancing Your Health and Beauty
Naturally 3
Benefitts of Ayurveda for Health and Beauty 3
Kapha Dosha: Characteristics and Imbalances 3
Determining Your Dominant Dosha 3
Determining Your Dominant Dosha 3
Determining Your Dominant Dosha 3

Ayurveda for Beginners: Enhancing Your Health and Beauty Naturally 3
Daily Routine (Dinacharya) for Optimal Health 3
Ayurvedic Diet and Nutrition 3
Ayurveda for Beginners: Enhancing Your Health and Beauty Naturally 3
Ayurvedic Detoxication (Panchakarma) 3
Balancing Emotions and Mental Well-being 3
Ayurveda for Beginners: Enhancing Your Health and Beauty Naturally 3
Ayurvedic Approach to Skincare 3
Ayurveda for Beginners: Enhancing Your Health and Beauty Naturally 3
Natural Ingredients for Healthy Skin 3
Ayurvedic Facial Treatments and Masks 3
Ayurveda for Beginners: Enhancing Your Health and Beauty Naturally 3
Hair Care and Scalp Treatments 3
Ayurvedic Beauty Rituals for Radiant Skin and Hair 3
Introduction to Ayurvedic Herbs 3
Common Ayurvedic Herbs for Health and Beauty 3
Preparing and Using Ayurvedic Herbal Remedies 3
Ayurveda for Beginners: Enhancing Your Health and Beauty Naturally 3
Herbal Remedies for Common Ailments 3
Ayurvedic Herbal Supplements and Formulations 3
Ayurveda for Beginners: Enhancing Your Health and Beauty Naturally 3
Ayurveda for Beginners: Enhancing Your Health and Beauty Naturally 3
Ayurvedic Approach to Stress and Anxiety 3
Ayurveda for Beginners: Enhancing Your Health and Beauty Naturally 3
Digestive Disorders and Ayurvedic Solutions 3
Ayurvedic Remedies for Skin Conditions 3
Women's Health and Ayurveda 3
Ayurveda for Weight Management 3
Ayurveda for Beginners: Enhancing Your Health and Beauty Naturally 3

- Ayurvedic Practices for Longevity ... 3
- Ayurvedic Anti-Aging Techniques ... 3
- Ayurveda for Beginners: Enhancing Your Health and Beauty Naturally ... 3
- Ayurvedic Herbs and Formulations for Anti-Aging ... 3
- Ayurvedic Practices for Maintaining Youthful Skin ... 3
- Ayurveda for Beginners: Enhancing Your Health and Beauty Naturally ... 3
- Mind-Body Practices for Aging Gracefully ... 3
- Creating a Personalized Ayurvedic Routine ... 3
- Ayurvedic Self-Care Practices for Busy Individuals ... 3
- Ayurvedic Tips for Healthy Relationships ... 3
- Ayurveda and Exercise ... 3
- Ayurvedic Practices for Better Sleep ... 3
- Recommended Books on Ayurveda ... 3
- Introduction To Ayurveda ... 1

Introduction to Ayurveda

Introduction To Ayurveda

What is Ayurveda ? Ayurveda, is ancient Indian system of medicine that has been practices by Indans for over 5000 years. The origins of Ayurveda can be traced back to the Vedas, the ancient scriptures of India. These texts contain knowledge on various subjects, including health, wellness, and longevity. Ayurveda, as a part of the Vedic tradition, evolved as a comprehensive system of medicine and healing, focusing on the balance of mind, body, and spirit. It has gained significant popularity in recent years because of its holistic approach to health and beauty.

One of its key principles is the copmprehensive understanding that each individual is unique and has a specific mind-body constitution, known as doshas. There are three main doshas: Vata, Pitta, and Kapha. These doshas govern various aspects of our physical and mental well-being. By identifying your dominant dosha, you can tailor your lifestyle, diet, and beauty practices.

Ayurveda helps restore balance, leading to improved overall health and radiant skin.

While Ayurveda offers valuable insights and techniques, it is important to consult a qualified Ayurvedic practitioner before implementing any practices. This ensures that the

individual needs and any underlying conditions are taken into account.

In conclusion, Ayurveda is a holistic system of medicine and beauty that promotes overall well-being by balancing the doshas and nurturing the mind, body, and spirit. By incorporating Ayurvedic practices into our daily lives, we can enhance our health and beauty naturally, leading to a more balanced and fulfilled Life

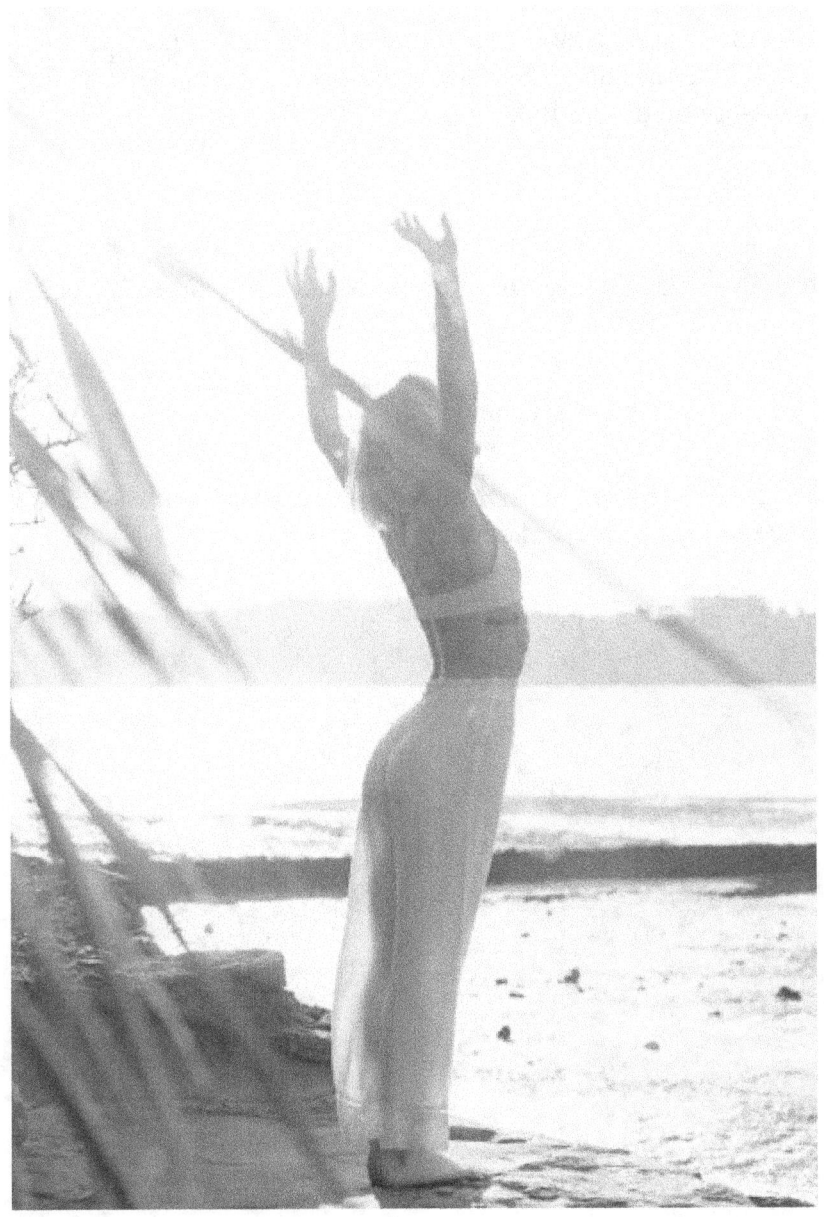

The following chapters delve into the rich history and underlying philosophy of Ayurveda, providing a comprehensive understanding of this time-honored tradition.

The word "Ayurveda" is derived from two Sanskrit words: "Ayur," meaning life, and "Veda," meaning knowledge. Thus,

Ayurveda can be translated as the

"science of life." This traditional system of medicine emphasizes the importance of preventive and curative measures to

maintain overall well-being.

Understanding and balancing these doshas is the key to achieving optimal health.

Ayurveda views health as a state of

harmony between the body, mind, and

spirit. It recognizes that imbalances in any aspect of life can lead to disease and

disharmony.

Therefore, Ayurvedic practices focus on restoring balance through lifestyle modifications, dietary choices, herbal remedies, and various therapeutic techniques.

History and Philosophy of Ayurveda

History and Philosopy of

Ayurveda

Ayurveda, is ancient Indian system of medicine that has been practices by

Indans for over 5000 years. The origins of Ayurveda can be traced back to the

Vedas, the ancient scriptures of India. These texts contain knowledge on various subjects, including health, wellness and longevity.

Ayurveda, as a part of the Vedic tradition, evolved as a comprehensive system of medicine and healing, focusing on the balance of mind, body, and spirit. It has gained significant popularity in recent years because of its holistic approach to health and beauty.

One of its key principles is the comprehensive understanding that each individual is unique and has a specific mind-body constitution, known as doshas.

There are three main doshas: Vata, Pitta, and Kapha. These doshas govern various aspects of our physical and mental well-being. By identifying your dominant dosha, you can tailor your lifestyle, diet, and beauty practices.

The History and the Philosphy of Ayurveda.

Ayurveda, as part of the Vedic tradition, evolved as a comprehensive system of medicines and healing, focusaing on the balance of mind, body and spirt.

Ayurvedic practices, such as Abhyanga (self-massage), Shirodhara (oil pouring on the forehead), and Panchakarma (cleansing therapies), have become widely recognized for their rejuvenating effects on the body and mind .

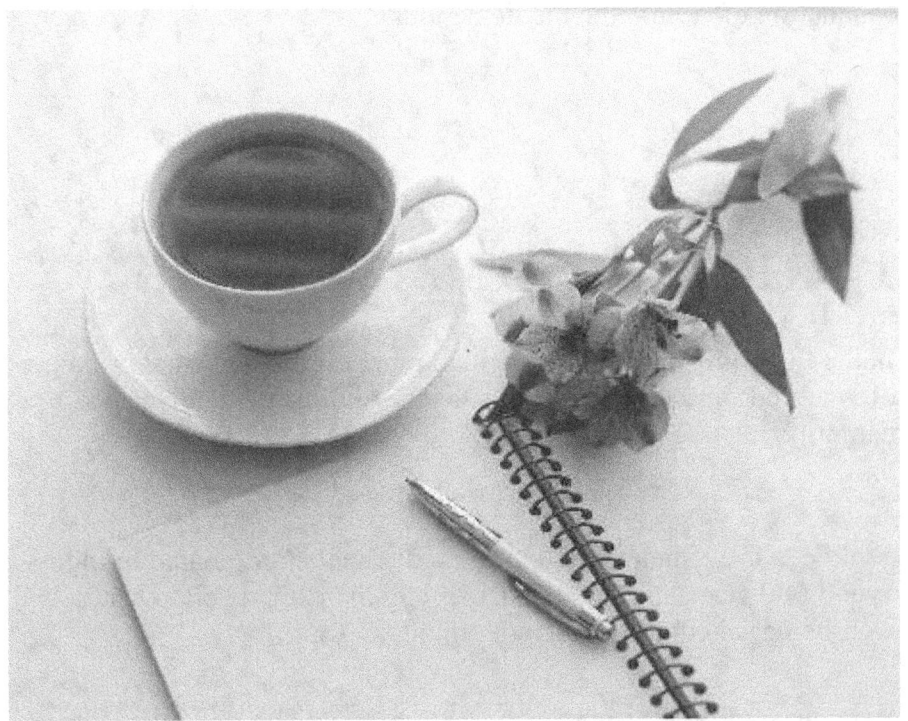

With its rich history and profound philosophy, Ayurveda offers a holistic approach to health and beauty that resonates with the needs of the modern world. By understanding the principles and practices of Ayurveda, individuals can enhance their well-being naturally and embark on a journey towards a healthier and more balanced life.

Throughout history, Ayurveda has undergone significant developments and refinements. This knowledge serves as the foundation of Ayurvedic medicine today.

Principles of Ayurveda

In the following chapters, we will explore the fundamental principles of Ayurveda and how they can enhance your health and beauty naturally.

Ayurveda is an ancient system of medicine that originated in India over 3,000 years ago. It emphasizes a holistic approach to health and well-being, integrating the body, mind, and spirit.

Here are some key principles of Ayurveda: **The Five Elements (Pancha Mahabhuta)**: Ayurveda is based on the concept that all matter is composed of five elements: earth (prithvi), water (apā), fire (tejas), air (vāyu), and ether (ākāśa). These elements combine to form the three doshas.

The Three Doshas: Doshas are the fundamental energies that govern physiological and psychological processes in the body.

The three doshas are: - **Vata** (air and ether): Governs movement and communication. - **Pitta** (fire and water): Governs digestion, metabolism, and energy production. - **Kapha** (earth and water): Governs structure, stability, and lubrication.
Each person has a unique combination of these doshas, known as their prakriti, which influences their physical and mental characteristics.

The Concept of Agni (Digestive Fire): Agni refers to the digestive fire or metabolic energy in the body. Proper digestion is considered crucial for health, and imbalances can lead to illness. Ayurveda emphasizes maintaining a healthy agni through diet, lifestyle, and herbal remedies.

The principles of Ayurveda offer a

holistic approach to health and beauty, focusing on achieving balance and

harmony within the body, mind, and spirit.

Detoxification and Rejuvenation:
Ayurveda promotes regular detoxification (panchakarma) to eliminate toxins (ama) from the body, restoring balance and promoting health. Rejuvenation therapies (rasayana) are also emphasized to support longevity and vitality.

Mind-Body Connection: Ayurveda recognizes the interconnectedness of the mind, body, and spirit. Mental and emotional health is seen as equally important as physical health, and practices such as meditation, yoga, and breathing exercises (pranayama) are integral to maintaining balance.

Diet and Nutrition: Ayurveda advocates for personalized diets based on an individual's dosha, season, and specific health needs. It emphasizes whole, natural foods and suggests balancing tastes (sweet, sour, salty, bitter, pungent, and astringent) for optimal health.

Lifestyle and Daily Routines (Dinacharya): Ayurveda endorses the importance of daily routines that align with natural rhythms (circadian rhythms) to promote balance. This includes practices like waking up early, maintaining a consistent meal schedule, and engaging in regular physical activity.

Seasonal Routines (Ritucharya): Ayurveda also emphasizes adapting lifestyle and dietary practices according to the seasons to maintain balance and health.

Holistic Healing: Ayurveda treats the root cause of illness rather than merely alleviating symptoms. It employs a range of treatments, including herbal medicine, dietary changes, yoga, meditation, and lifestyle modifications.

Individualization: Ayurveda recognizes that each individual is unique, and treatments should be tailored to the individual's specific constitution, imbalances, and life circumstances. By integrating these principles, Ayurveda aims to promote harmony within the body and mind, leading to optimal health and well-being.

Ayurveda recognizes the close connection between the mind and body. It emphasizes the importance of maintaining mental and emotional balance for overall health and beauty

Practices such as meditation, yoga, and breathing exercises can help reduce stress, improve mental clarity, and enhance your natural beauty.

The principles of Ayurveda offer a holistic approach to health and beauty. By

understanding your dosha, maintaining a strong digestive fire, eliminating toxins, and nurturing your mind and body, you can enhance your health and beauty naturally.

By incorporating Ayurvedic practices into your daily routine can lead to a harmonious and balanced life, promoting overall well-being and radiating beauty from within.

Ayurvedic practices such as eating mindfully, avoiding overeating, and consuming foods that are appropriate for your dosha can help enhance digestion and promote overall well-being.

Ayurveda also emphasizes the concept of ama, which refers to toxins that accumulate in the body due to poor digestion and lifestyle choices. Ama is believed to be the root cause of many health and beauty issues.

Ayurvedic practices such as detoxification, known as Panchakarma, and incorporating herbs and spices with detoxifying properties can help eliminate ama and restore balance to the body.

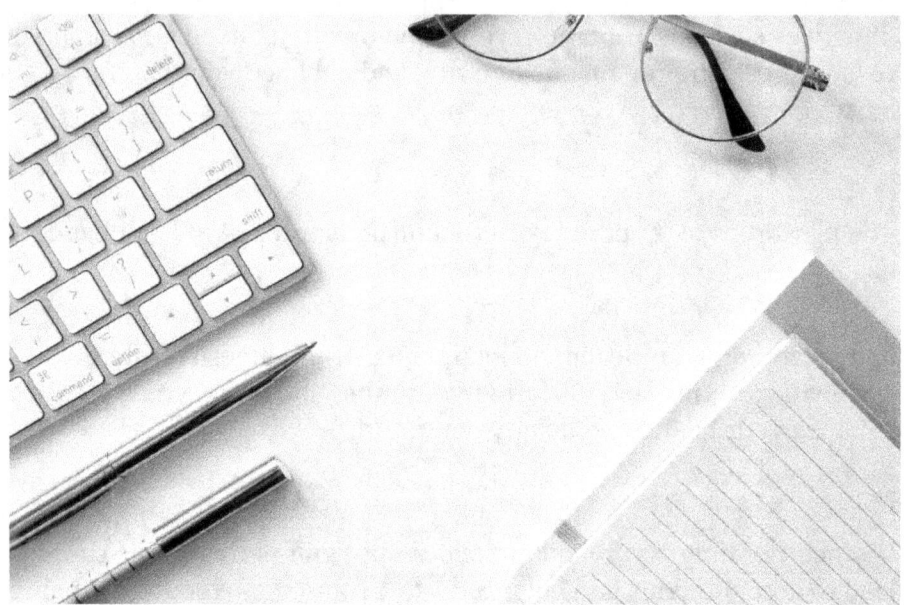

Another benefit of Ayurveda is its recognition of individual uniqueness. Unlike many

modern beauty practices that adopt a one-size-fits-all approach, Ayurveda acknowledges that each person is unique and requires personalized care. By understanding your specific constitution and skin type, Ayurveda helps tailor treatments and skincare routines that address your specific needs, resulting in a more effective and personalized approach to

health and beauty.

Ayurveda promotes a healthy lifestyle that includes proper nutrition, regular exercise, and stress management. These practices not only contribute to overall well-being but also

have a direct impact on the skin's health and appearance.

By following Ayurvedic dietary guidelines and engaging in activities that promote balance and relaxation, individuals can experience improved digestion, reduced inflammation, and a natural glow from within.

Embracing Ayurveda for Enhanced Health and Beauty

Welcome to the world of Ayurveda, the ancient healing system that has been practiced for thousands of years. In this chapter, we will embark on a journey to explore the wonders of Ayurvedic health and beauty practices.

Whether you are completely new to Ayurveda or have some prior knowledge, this chapter will serve as a comprehensive guide to enhance your health and beauty naturally.

Ayurveda, meaning "the science of life," is a holistic approach to well-being that focuses on balancing the mind, body, and spirit. Unlike modern medicine, Ayurveda treats the root cause of imbalances rather than just alleviating symptoms.

By harmonizing the body's energies, known as doshas – Vata, Pitta, and Kapha – Ayurveda

helps restore and maintain optimal health.

To begin your Ayurvedic journey, it's essential to understand your unique dosha constitution.

This can be through a series of assessments, including observing your physical attributes, personality traits, and even your digestion and sleep.

Ayurveda, offers an array of natural remedies and practices to enhance both health and beauty. With its holistic approach, Ayurveda focuses on achieving balance and harmony within the body, mind, and spirit

In this chapter, we will explore the key

principles of Ayurveda and how they can be incorporated into your daily routine to enhance your overall well-being and radiance.

One of the fundamental principles of Ayurveda is the concept of doshas.

According to Ayurveda, each individual possesses a unique combination of the three doshas – Vata, Pitta, and Kapha – which govern various physiological and psychological functions. Understanding your predominant dosha can

help you tailor your health and beauty practices to achieve optimal results.

Ayurveda advocates the importance of a healthy diet for maintaining good health and promoting natural beauty. By incorporating Ayurvedic principles into your eating habits,

such as favoring fresh, seasonal, and organic foods and avoiding processed and refined ingredients, you can nourish your body from within and achieve a radiant complexion.

In addition to a balanced diet, Ayurveda emphasizes the importance of daily self-care rituals, known as Dinacharya.

These rituals include practices such as tongue scraping, oil pulling, dry brushing, and self-massage with herbal oils.

By incorporating these practices into your daily routine, you can promote detoxification, improve circulation, and enhance the health and vitality of your skin and hair.

Determing your dominant Dosha

One of the primary benefits of Ayurveda is its focus on balancing the body's three doshas – Vata, Pitta, and Kapha.

Imbalances in these doshas can lead to various health issues and skin problems. By identifying your dominant dosha and making the necessary lifestyle and dietary adjustments, Ayurveda helps restore balance, leading to improved overall health and radiant skin.

While Ayurveda offers valuable insights and techniques, it is important to consult a qualified Ayurvedic practitioner before implementing any practices.

This ensures that the recommendations are tailored to individual needs and any underlying conditions are taken into account.

Ayurveda offers a holistic approach to achieving balance in our lives by recommending personalized lifestyle modifications, dietary choices, herbal remedies, and self-care rituals tailored to each dosha.

By understanding our dosha it allows us to make informed choices regarding our health and beauty practices.

A principle of Ayurveda is the importance of maintaining a strong digestive fire, known as Agni.

According to Ayurveda, a healthy digestion is the cornerstone of good health and beauty.

We will delve deeper into each dosha, exploring how they influence our physical and emotional well-being. We will discover practical and effective Ayurvedic practices that can enhance our health and beauty naturally.

By delving deeper into each dosha and exploring how they influence our

physical and emotional well-being we can discover practical and effective Ayurvedic practices that can enhance our health and beauty naturally, helping us achieve a harmonious state of

being.

Whether you are new to Ayurveda or already familiar with itsprinciples, this book aims to empower you with the knowledge and tools to incorporate Ayurvedic health and beauty practices into your daily life. By embracing this ancient wisdom, you can unlock the secrets to lasting health, radiant beauty, and overall well-being.

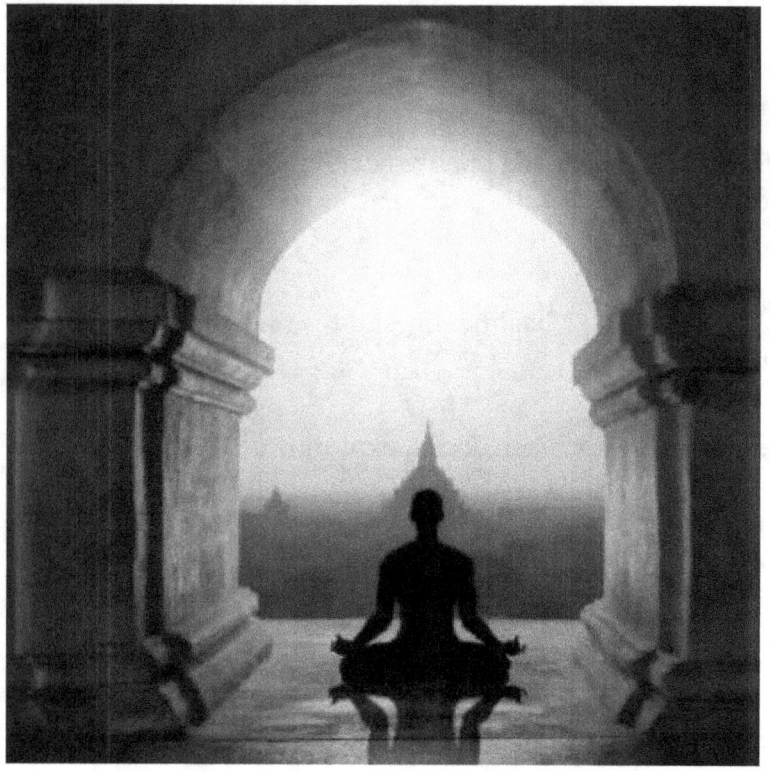

Vata Dosha: Characteristics and Imbalances

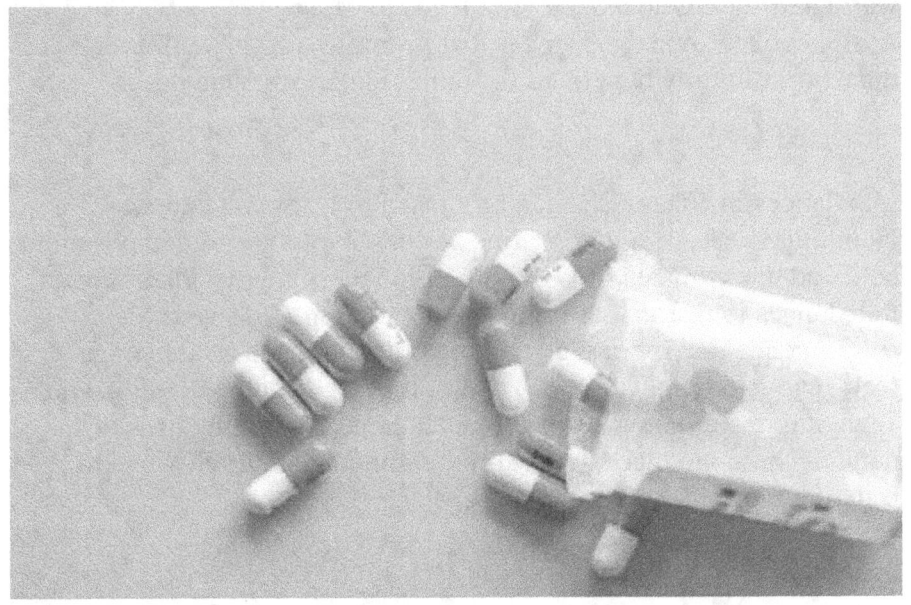

Characteristics of Vata Dosha:
Vata dosha is characterized by certain qualities that reflect its elemental nature. These qualities include dryness, lightness, coldness, and mobility. Individuals with a dominant Vata dosha tend to have a slender frame, dry skin and hair, and a restless mind. They often have a creative and enthusiastic nature, displaying quick thinking and adaptability.

Imbalances in Vata Dosha: When Vata dosha becomes imbalanced, it can lead to various physical and emotional issues. Common symptoms of Vata imbalance include dry skin, constipation, insomnia, anxiety, and joint pain. As Vata governs movement, an excess of this dosha can cause excessive movement in the body, leading to restlessness, nervousness, and even insomnia.

One of the key aspects of balancing Vata dosha is establishing a regular routine. This includes maintaining consistent meal times, sleep patterns, and exercise routines. It is also important to keep warm and stay hydrated, as Vata tends to cause dryness. Consuming warm, cooked foods and spices that promote warmth and improve digestion is highly beneficial for individuals with Vata dosha.

Imbalances in Vata dosha can be caused by various factors, including stress, irregular routines, excessive travel, and exposure to cold and dry climates. It is important to identify and address these imbalances to restore harmony and well-being. Ayurveda also recommends incorporating self-care practices such as abhyanga (self-massage with warm oil), practicing yoga and meditation, and engaging in calming activities like reading or spending time in nature. These practices help calm the mind and nourish the body, bringing balance to Vata dosha.

Balancng Vata Dosa:
By understanding the characteristics and imbalances of Vata dosha, you can make conscious choices to enhance your health and beauty naturally. By adopting Ayurvedic health and beauty practices tailored to your unique constitution, you can restore balance, promote vitality, and experience a state of holistic well-being.

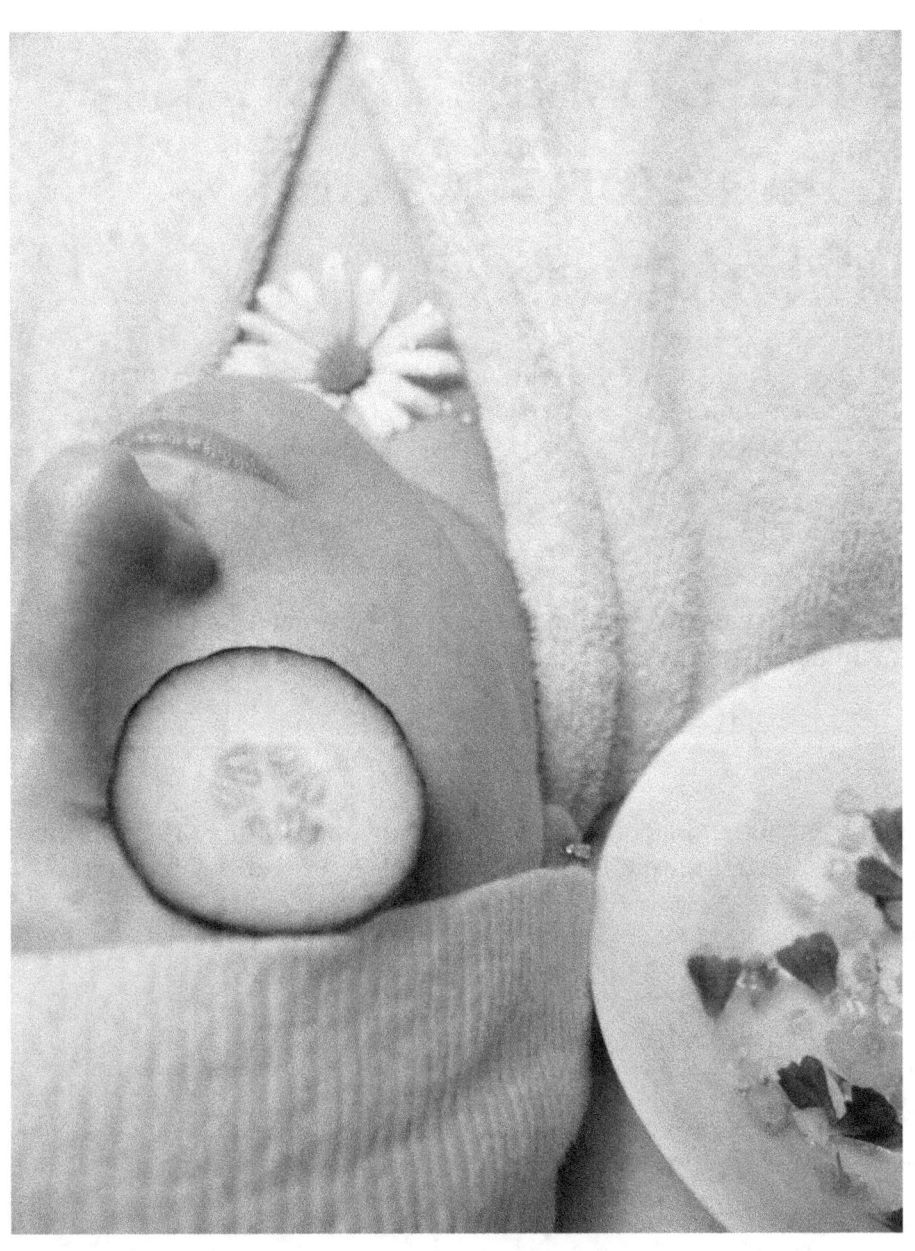

Pitta Dosha: Characteristics and Imbalances

In the ancient science of Ayurveda, one of the essential concepts is the understanding

of doshas, or the three fundamental energies that govern our bodies and minds. Pitta

dosha, the energy of fire and water, plays a crucial role in maintaining our overall health and beauty.

Understanding the characteristics and imbalances of Pitta dosha can help us make informed choices to enhance our well-being naturally.

Characteristics of Pitta Dosha

Pitta dosha is responsible for our metabolism, digestion, and transformation. Individuals with a dominant Pitta dosha tend to have a

medium build, sharp intellect, and intense focus. They are often dynamic, ambitious, and possess a strong determination. Pitta individuals are also known for their strong

digestion and appetite, as well as their radiant skin and lustrous hair.

However, when Pitta dosha becomes imbalanced, it can lead to various health and

beauty issues. Excess Pitta can manifest as anger, irritability, and impatience. Physically, it may cause inflammation, excessive heat, and sensitivity to the sun. Imbalanced Pitta can also result in skin conditions like acne, rashes, and premature graying of hair.

To balance Pitta dosha, Ayurveda recommends adopting a cooling and calming lifestyle. This includes maintaining a regular routine, practicing mindfulness, and engaging in activities that promote relaxation and stress reduction, such as yoga and meditation.

A Pitta-pacifying diet emphasizes the consumption of cooling foods like fresh fruits, vegetables, and herbs, while minimizing spicy, oily, and processed foods.

Imbalances of Pitta Dosha:
Additionally, Ayurveda suggests specific herbs and treatments to address Pitta imbalances. Aloe vera, coriander, and rose are known for their cooling properties and can be used in skincare routines to soothe inflamed skin. Ayurvedic therapies like

Shirodhara, where a gentle stream of oil is poured over the forehead, can help calm the mind and balance Pitta.

Balancing Pitta Dosha:
By understanding the characteristics and imbalances of Pitta dosha, we can make conscious choices to restore balance and enhance our health and beauty naturally.

Embracing Ayurvedic principles and practices can help us lead a more harmonious life, where our inner fire is balanced, and our radiant beauty shines through.

Kapha Dosha: Characteristics and Imbalances

Kapha Dosha is primarily composed of the earth and water elements, making it inherently stable, solid, and cool.

Individuals with dominant Kapha tend to have a robust physique, lustrous skin, and a calm and serene disposition. They often possess qualities like endurance, strength, and resilience. Kapha types are known for their nurturing and compassionate nature, making them excellent caretakers and friends.

Imbalances of Kapa Dosha:
However, when Kapha Dosha becomes imbalanced, it can manifest in various physical and emotional symptoms. Excessive Kapha can lead to a feeling of heaviness and sluggishness in the body, causing weight gain, water retention, and slow digestion. Imbalanced Kapha can also lead to respiratory issues, such as congestion, allergies, and excessive mucus production. On an emotional level, Kapha imbalances may result in feelings of attachment, possessiveness, and resistance to change. Mental fog, lethargy, and a lack of motivation are also common signs of excessive Kapha.

Understanding these imbalances is crucial as it allows us to address them proactively and restore balance to our mind, body, and spirit.

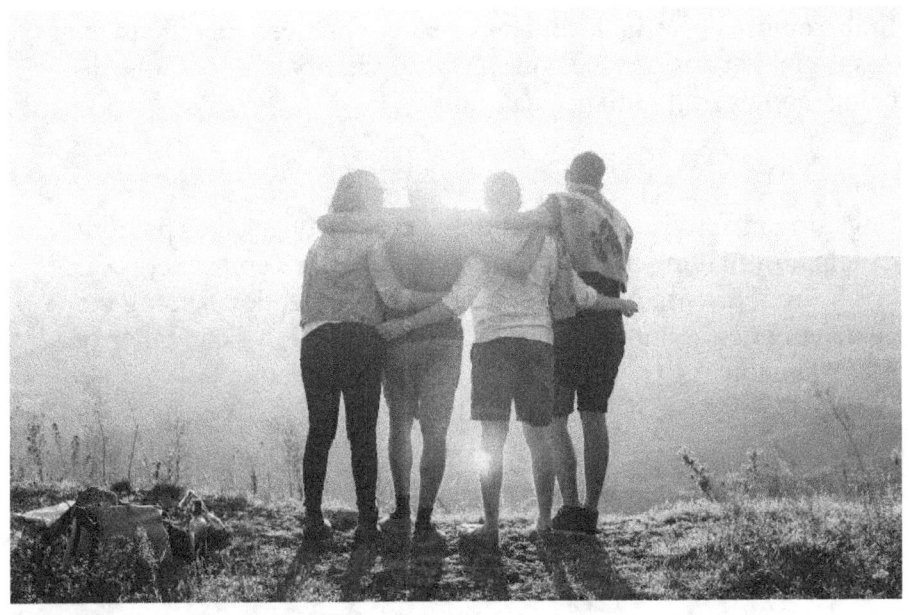

Balancing Kapha Doha:
To bring Kapha Dosha back into equilibrium, Ayurveda offers various holistic practices. Regular exercise, particularly activities that are vigorous and stimulating, can help balance the heaviness associated with excessive Kapha.

Incorporating a variety of spices and herbs, such as ginger, turmeric, and cinnamon, into our diet can enhance digestion and metabolism, reducing Kapha's dominance. Furthermore, adopting a daily self-care routine that includes dry brushing, warm oil massages, and stimulating essential oils like rosemary and eucalyptus can invigorate the senses and promote a sense of lightness.

Engaging in activities that encourage creativity, such as painting, dancing, or playing music, can also help uplift Kapha energy and bring about a sense of joy and inspiration. By understanding the characteristics and imbalances of Kapha Dosha, we can tailor our lifestyle choices to promote balance and well-being.

Embracing Ayurvedic health and beauty practices specific to our dosha can help us enhance our physical vitality, emotional well-being, and overall radiance naturally.

Engaging in activities that encourage creativity, such as painting, dancing, or playing music, can also help uplift Kapha energy and bring about a sense of joy and inspiration. By understanding the characteristics and imbalances of Kapha Dosha, we can tailor our lifestyle choices to promote balance and well-being.
Embracing Ayurvedic health and beauty practices specific to our dosha can help us enhance our physical vitality, emotional well-being, and overall radiance naturally.

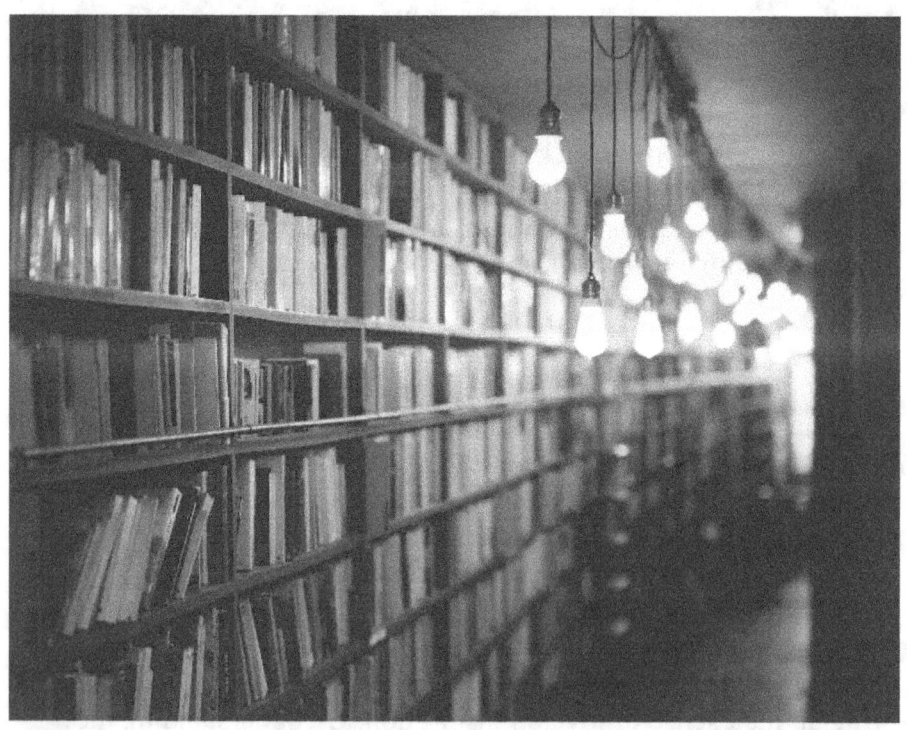

Daily Routine (Dinacharya) for Optimal Health

In the fast-paced world we live in

today, it can be challenging to prioritize our health and well-being. However,

incorporating a daily routine

(dinacharya) into our lives is crucial for achieving optimal health. Ayurveda, the ancient Indian system of medicine,

offers valuable insights and practices that can help us enhance our overall well-being and beauty naturally.

The daily routine in Ayurveda is

designed to harmonize our mind, body, and spirit. By aligning ourselves with

the natural rhythms of the day, we can promote balance, vitality, and longevity.

Let's explore some Ayurvedic health and beauty practices that you can

incorporate into your daily routine:

1. Rise with the Sun: Waking up early in the morning, preferably before sunrise, is considered essential in Ayurveda.

This time is known as brahma muhurta, the most auspicious time for spiritual practices. It allows us to connect with the stillness and silence of the early morning, setting the tone for a peaceful and productive day.

2. Tongue Scraping: Upon waking, gently scrape your tongue with a copper tongue scraper. This simple practice helps remove toxins (ama) that have accumulated overnight and promotes oral hygiene, fresh breath, and proper digestion.

3. Oil Pulling: Swish a tablespoon of

organic sesame or coconut oil in your mouth for 10-15 minutes. This ancient practice, known as oil pulling, detoxifies the oral cavity, improves oral health, and

can even contribute to overall well-being.

4. Self-Massage Abhyanga): Before showering, indulge in a self-massage

using warm oil. This traditional practice helps nourish the skin, improve

suitable for your dosha Ayurvedic mind- body type) to enhance the benefits.

5. Eat Mindfully: Enjoy a nourishing breakfast that includes a balance of all six tastes –sweet, sour, salty, bitter, pungent, and astringent. Ayurveda emphasizes the

importance of mindful eating, savoring each bite, and choosing fresh, seasonal, and locally sourced ingredients.

6. Yoga and Meditation: Engage in a regular yoga and meditation practice to cultivatephysical strength, flexibility, mental clarity, and emotional balance. These practices help

reduce stress, enhance vitality, and promote overall well-being.

7. Early Dinner: Have an early, light dinner at three hours before bedtime. This allows for proper digestion and ensures a restful sleep.

Remember, consistency is key when incorporating these practices into your daily routine. Start with small steps and gradually build upon them. Ayurveda teaches us that true beauty and optimal health come from within, and by embracing this ancient wisdom, you can enhance your overall wellbeing naturally.

Disclaimer: The content provided here is for informational purposes only and should not be considered medical advice. Please consult with a qualified healthcare professional

before incorporating any Ayurvedic practices into your daily routine.

Ayurvedic Diet and Nutrition

In today's fast-paced world, it's easy to neglect our health and beauty. We often find ourselves reaching for quick and convenient meals that do little to nourish our bodies.

However, Ayurveda, offers a holistic approach to health and beauty that focuses on balancing the mind, body, and spirit. Central to this approach is the Ayurvedic diet and nutrition, which plays a vital role in promoting overall well-being.

The Ayurvedic diet is based on the belief that each individual has a unique constitution, or dosha, which determines their physical and mental characteristics.

There are three primary doshas: Vata, Pitta, and Kapha. By understanding our dosha, we can tailor our diet to meet our specific needs and achieve optimal health.

For those with a Vata constitution, which is characterized by qualities such as coldness, dryness, and lightness, a diet that includes warm, nourishing foods is recommended.

This may include cooked grains, root vegetables, and healthy fats like ghee or sesame oil. Pitta individuals, who tend to have a fiery nature, should focus on cooling and

hydrating foods such as fresh fruits, leafy greens, and coconut water.

As for Kapha individuals, who are often heavier and more grounded, a diet that emphasizes light, dry, and spicy foods is beneficial. This may involve incorporating legumes, bitter greens,and warming spices like ginger and cinnamon.

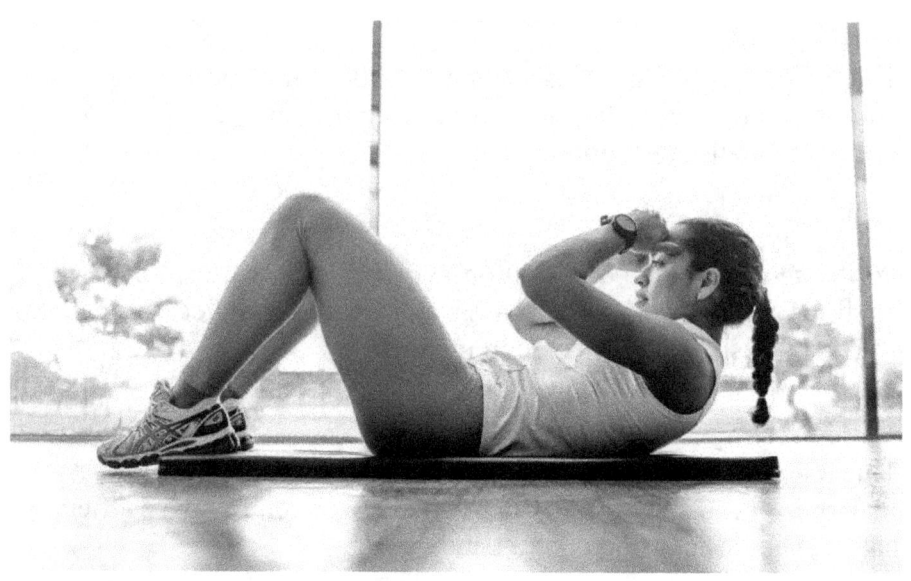

In addition to considering our dosha, Ayurveda also emphasizes the importance of mindful eating. This means being fully present and aware while enjoying our meals, chewing our food thoroughly, and avoiding distractions. This practice promotes better digestion and

nutrient absorption, leading to improved overall health.

Furthermore, Ayurveda encourages the consumption of fresh, seasonal, and locally

sourced foods. This ensures that we are consuming foods that are in harmony with our

environment and provides us with the necessary nutrients to support our well-being. It also emphasizes the importance of a balanced diet that includes all six tastes: sweet, sour, salty, bitter, pungent, and astringent. Each taste has specific effects on the body and helps to maintain equilibrium.

By adopting an Ayurvedic diet and nutrition plan, we can enhance our health and beauty naturally. It is a personalized approach that recognizes the unique needs of our body and mind. So, let us embrace this ancient wisdom and embark on a journey towards optimal well-being, where nourishing our bodies becomes a way of life.

Importance of Proper Digestion (Agni)

In the ancient science of Ayurveda, digestion, or Agni, is considered the foundation of good

health and beauty. It is believed that a strong and balanced Agni is essential for the efficient functioning of our body and mind.

Ayurvedic health and beauty practices have long emphasized the significance of proper digestion, recognizing its role in promoting overall well-being and enhancing our natural beauty.

One of the key reasons why proper digestion is essential is that it allows our body to extract the maximum benefits from the food we eat.

No matter how healthy our diet is, if our Agni is weak, we may not be able to fully absorb the nutrients, vitamins, and minerals present in our meals. This can lead to nutrient

deficiencies, weakened immune system, and various health complications.

Moreover, Ayurveda teaches us that a healthy digestive system is intricately connected to our emotional well-being.

According to this ancient wisdom, our gut is considered the "second brain" as it

produces neurotransmitters that influence our mood and emotions. When our digestion is impaired, it can lead to imbalances in these neurotransmitters, resulting in mood swings, anxiety, andeven depression.

Ayurvedic health and beauty practices emphasize the importance of nurturing our Agni through mindful eating habits and lifestyle choices.

This includes consuming fresh, whole foods that are suitable for our unique body type,

incorporating spices and herbs that aid digestion, and avoiding processed and heavy foods that burden the digestive system.

Ayurvedic Detoxication (Panchakarma)

In the quest for a healthier and more balanced lifestyle, many individuals are turning to Ayurvedic practices to enhance their overall well-being. Ayurveda, the ancient Indian

system of medicine, offers a holistic approach to health and beauty that focuses on restoring balance and harmony within the body.

One of the key techniques used in Ayurveda to achieve this balance is known as Panchakarma, a detoxification process that eliminates toxins and rejuvenates the body and mind.

Panchakarma, which translates to "five actions," is a comprehensive detoxification method that targets the root causes of imbalances in the body. It involves a series of five therapeutic procedures, each designed to cleanse and restore specific bodily systems.

These procedures include Vamana (therapeutic vomiting), Virechana (purgation), Basti (enema), Nasya (nasal administration), and Raktamokshana (bloodletting). These procedures are performed under the guidance of a trained Ayurvedic practitioner who tailors the treatment to individual needs.

The primary goal of Panchakarma is to remove accumulated toxins, known as Ama, from

the body. Ama is formed due to poor digestion, improper lifestyle choices, and

environmental factors. When Ama accumulates in the body, it disrupts the natural balance of the doshas Vata, Pitta, and Kapha) and impairs the functioning of various organs and systems.

Panchakarma helps to eliminate Ama from the body, allowing the doshas to return to their natural state and promoting optimal health.

Panchakarma offers numerous benefits for both physical and mental well-being. It improves digestion, boosts the immune system, enhances mental clarity, and promotes a sense of

nd promotes a sense of rejuvenation and vitality.

It can also help with weight management, skin disorders, allergies, and chronic conditions such as arthritis and asthma.

Additionally, Panchakarma is known to reduce stress, anxiety, and fatigue, providing a deep sense of relaxation and overall balance.

It is important to note that Panchakarma is a specialized procedure that should only be performed under the guidance of a qualified Ayurvedic practitioner. The treatment plan is tailored to suit each individual's unique constitution and health needs. Prior to undergoing

Panchakarma, a thorough assessment is conducted to determine the doshic imbalances and create a personalized treatment protocol.

In conclusion, Panchakarma is a powerful Ayurvedic detoxification process that

offers a holistic approach to health and beauty.

By eliminating toxins and restoring balance within the body, it promotes By eliminating toxins and restoring balance within the body, it promotes overall wellness and rejuvenation

If you are seeking a natural and effective method to enhance your health and beauty,

Panchakarma could be the perfect solution for you. Consult with an experienced Ayurvedic

practitioner to embark on this transformative journey towards optimal well-being.

Balancing Emotions and Mental Well-being

Understanding the Mind-Body Connection:

According to Ayurveda, our emotions are closely linked to our physical health. An imbalance in one can lead to disturbances in the other. For instance, chronic stress can manifest as physical symptoms like headaches, digestive issues, or even skin problems.

Therefore, achieving emotional balance is crucial for optimal health and beauty. Ayurvedic Practices for Emotional Balance.

1. Self-Awareness: The first step in balancing emotions is to develop self- awareness. Understanding your emotional triggers, recognizing

negative patterns, and practicing mindfulness can

help you respond to situations in a more balanced manner.

2. Daily Routine: Following a disciplined daily routine, known as dinacharya, isessential for maintaining emotional well-being. This includes waking up early, practicing meditation or deep breathing exercises, and engaging in physical

activities like yoga or walking.

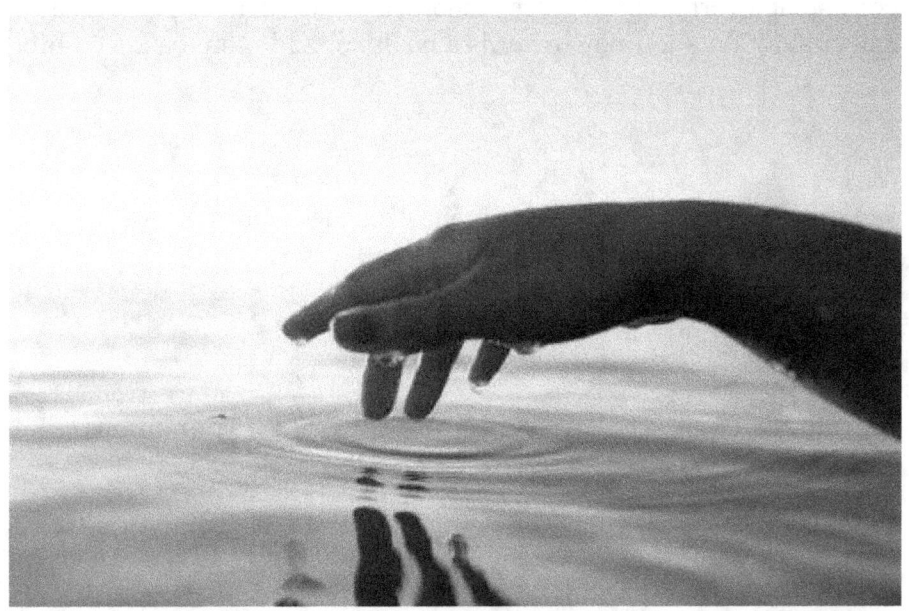

3. Herbal Remedies: Ayurveda offers a wide range of herbal remedies to support emotional well-being. Adaptogenic herbs like Ashwagandha and Brahmi can helpreduce stress and anxiety. Additionally, herbs such as Tulsi and Jatamansi have a calming effect on the mind.

4. Aromatherapy: The use of essential oils is an effective Ayurvedic practice tobalance emotions. Oils like lavender, rose, and chamomile can help calm the mind and promote relaxation. Incorporating aromatherapy into your daily routine through diffusers, massages, or

inhaling directly can have a positive impact on your mental well-being.

By incorporating these Ayurvedic practices into your daily life, you can enhance your emotional balance and promote mental well-being. Remember, emotional health is an ongoing process that requires consistent effort and self- care. Embrace the wisdom of Ayurveda and embark on a journey towards a healthier and more balanced life.

5. Nourishing Diet: Ayurveda emphasizes the importance of a healthy diet for emotional balance.

Consuming fresh, whole foods that are suitable for your unique constitution can help nourish both the body and mind.

Avoiding processed foods, excessive caffeine, and alcohol is also recommended.

In today's fast-paced world, maintaining emotional balance and mental well-being has become increasingly challenging.

Stress, anxiety, and other emotional imbalances can significantly impact our overall health and beauty. Ayurveda, an ancient holistic healing system, offers profound insights and practices to help restore harmony and promote emotional well-being.

Ayurvedic Approach to Skincare

Ayurvedic Skincare and Beauty Rituals

Skincare is an essential part of our daily routine, but have you ever considered adopting an Ayurvedic approach to enhance your beauty naturally? In this subchapter, we will explore

the ancient wisdom of Ayurveda and how it can transform your skincare routine into a holistic and rejuvenating experience.

Ayurveda believes that true beauty comes from within. It emphasizes the importance of balance and harmony between the mind, body, and spirit to achieve overall wellness. Therefore, Ayurvedic skincare practices not only focus on external treatments but also emphasize internal nourishment and self-care rituals.

One of the fundamental principles of Ayurveda is the recognition of different skin types or doshas - Vata, Pitta, and Kapha. Each dosha has specific characteristics and requires a

unique approach to skincare. Understanding your dosha can help you tailor your skincare routine to address your specific needs and achieve optimal results.

Ayurvedic skincare starts with cleansing, using natural ingredients such as rose water,

honey, or herbal powders. These gentle cleansers remove impurities without stripping the skin of its natural oils.

Followed by cleansing, Ayurveda recommends exfoliating to remove dead skin cells and promote cell regeneration. Natural exfoliants like oatmeal, sandalwood, or chickpea flour can be used according to your dosha.

After cleansing and exfoliating, Ayurveda encourages the use of herbal face masks to nourish and rejuvenate the skin. These masks are made from a combination of Ayurvedic herbs, clays, and oils, carefully selected to suit your dosha.

Applying these masks regularly can help balance your dosha and improve the overall

health and appearance of your skin. Ayurveda also places great importance on facial massage or Abhyanga.

This technique stimulates the circulation, detoxifies the skin, and promotes a radiant complexion. Using warm herbal oils specific to your dosha, gently massage your face in circular motions, paying attention to pressure points and areas of tension. This self-care ritual not only enhances your skin's health but also provides a calming and rejuvenating experience for the mind and spirit.

In addition to external practices, Ayurveda emphasizes the importance of nourishing your skin from within. A balanced diet, rich in fresh fruits, vegetables, and whole grains, along with proper hydration, is essential for maintaining healthy skin. Ayurvedic herbs and supplements, such as turmeric, neem, and amla, can also support skin health and beauty from the inside out.

By adopting Ayurvedic principles in your skincare routine, you can experience the transformative power of natural ingredients and self-care rituals.

Embracing this holistic approach to skincare will not only enhance your external beauty but also promote overall health and well-being. So, take a step towards Ayurveda and unlock the secrets of radiant and naturally beautiful skin.

Natural Ingredients for Healthy Skin

When it comes to achieving healthy and radiant skin, many of us turn to expensive skincare products that promise

miraculous results.

However, what if we told you that the key to unlocking your skin's true potential lies in the power of nature? Ayurveda, is an ancient Indian system of medicine and wellness.

It offers a treasure trove of natural ingredients that can nourish, rejuvenate, and

enhance your skin's health and beauty.

In this chapter, we will explore some of the most potent and widely used natural ingredients in Ayurvedic health and beauty practices. These ingredients are easily accessible, affordable, and free from harmful chemicals that can often be found in commercial skincare products.

By incorporating these natural wonders into your skincare routine, you can harness their therapeutic properties and achieve a healthy glow from within.

One of the most revered ingredients in Ayurveda is aloe vera. With its soothing and cooling properties, aloe vera is an excellent remedy for various skin conditions,

including acne, sunburns, and dryness. Its gel-like substance is rich in vitamins,

minerals, and antioxidants, which help to moisturize and heal the skin, leaving it soft and supple.

Another Ayurvedic gem is turmeric, a spice that has been used for centuries in Indian cuisine and skincare. Turmeric's active compound, curcumin, possesses powerful anti- inflammatory and antioxidant properties, making it a great ally for combating skin inflammation, hyperpigmentation, and signs of aging.

Incorporating turmeric into face masks or consuming it orally can result in a brighter and more youthful complexion.

In addition to aloe vera and turmeric, Ayurveda also emphasizes the use of neem, rose water, and sandalwood for healthy skin.

Neem, known as nature's pharmacy, possesses antibacterial properties that can help with acne-prone skin.

Rose water, derived from rose petals, acts as a natural toner, hydrating and refreshing the skin.

Sandalwood, with its pleasant aroma and cooling effect, can soothe and rejuvenate tired and irritated skin.

By incorporating these natural ingredients into your daily skincare routine, you can harness the power of Ayurveda to enhance your skin's health and beauty naturally.

Remember, Ayurveda is not just about external treatments but also focuses on maintaining

internal balance through a healthy diet, lifestyle, and mindfulness practices. So, take a step towards holistic skincare and embrace the beauty of nature for a radiant and glowing complexion.

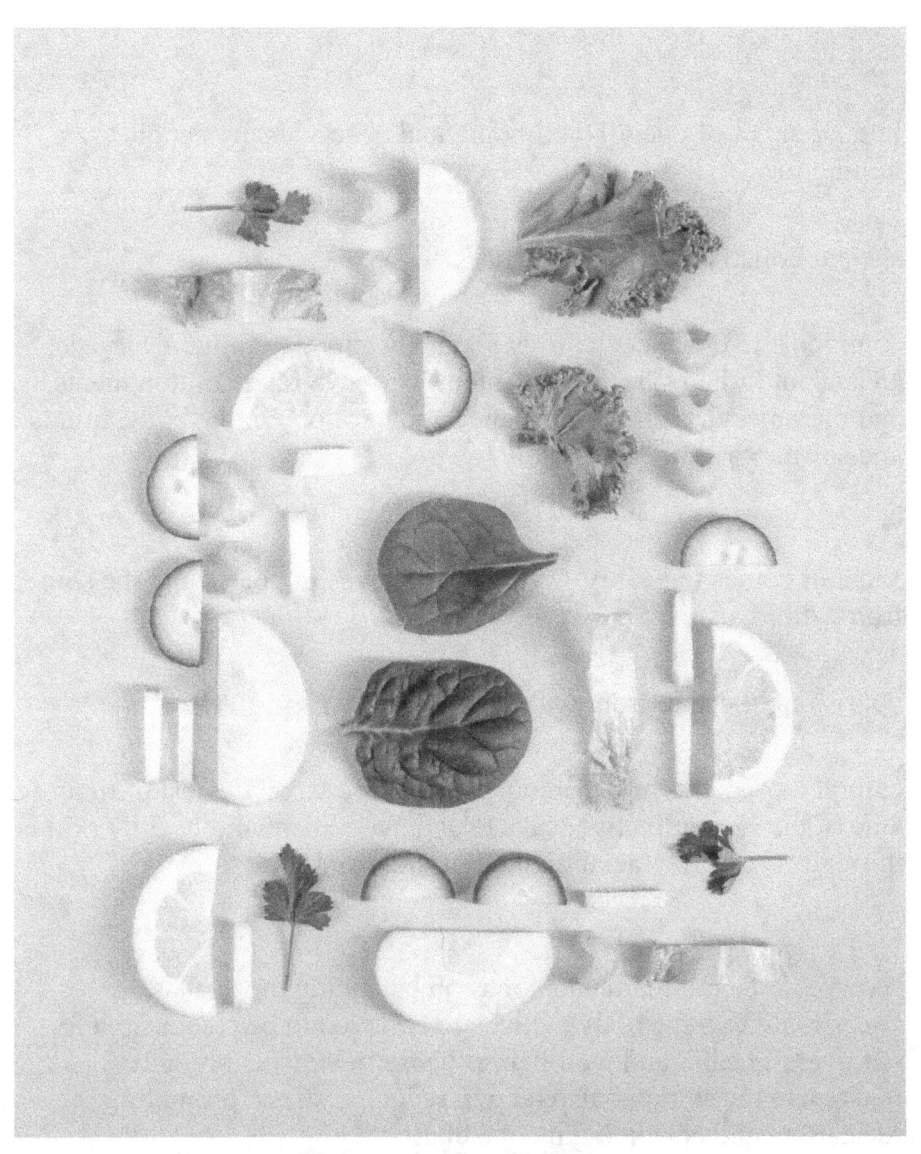

Ayurvedic Facial Treatments and Face Masks

In the pursuit of overall well-being and beauty, many people are turning to

ancient holistic practices, such as

Ayurveda, to enhance their health and beauty naturally. Ayurveda, an ancient Indian system of medicine, offers a range of treatments and therapies that promote balance and harmony in the body, mind, and spirit.

When it comes to beauty, Ayurveda believes in nourishing the skin from within, using

nourishing the skin from within, using

natural ingredients and techniques that have stood the test of time. One of the most effective ways to achieve radiant and healthy skin is through Ayurvedic facial treatments and masks.

Ayurvedic facial treatments focus on balancing the doshas, or energies, within the body, which are believed to be responsible for our overall health and well-being. These treatments not only rejuvenate the skin but also help in reducing stress, promoting relaxation, and enhancing mental clarity.

Ayurvedic facials often involve a combination of massage, herbal steam, and the application of specific herbal and natural ingredients tailored to an individual's unique dosha type.

One popular Ayurvedic facial treatment is the use of herbal steam to cleanse and detoxify

the skin. This involves placing the face over a steaming pot of water infused with herbs such as neem, tulsi, or rosemary. The steam opens up the pores, allowing the herbs to penetrate deep into the skin, cleansing and purifying it.

rosemary.

This treatment not only removes impurities but also improves blood circulation, resulting in a healthy and radiant complexion.

Ayurvedic facial masks are another key component of these treatments. These masks are formulated using natural ingradients. such as turmeric, sandalwood, honey, and a variety of herbs and spices.

Each ingredient is carefully chosen for its specific properties to address various skin concerns. For instance, a turmeric mask is often used to brighten the skin and reduce inflammation, while a sandalwood mask is known for its cooling and calming effects.

Regular use of Ayurvedic facial masks can help in improving skin texture, reducing blemishes, and achieving a natural glow.

These masks nourish and hydrate the skin, providing it with essential nutrients and antioxidants, which are vital for maintaining its health and youthfulness.

In conclusion, Ayurvedic facial treatments and masks offer a holistic and natural approach to skincare. By focusing on balancing the energies within the body and using nourishing ingredients, these treatments can improve the health and beauty of your skin.

Whether you are seeking relaxation, rejuvenation, or a natural way to enhance your beauty, Ayurvedic facials are a wonderful addition to your health and beauty routine. Embrace the wisdom of Ayurveda and experience the transformative power of these ancient practices.

Hair Care and Scalp Treatments

In the quest for overall health and beauty, it is essential not to neglect our crowning glory – our hair. In Ayurveda, hair care and scalp treatments are considered integral parts of

maintaining a balanced and holistic approach to wellness.

This chapter explores the various Ayurvedic techniques and remedies that can enhance the

health and beauty of your hair naturally.

Ayurvedic hair care begins with understanding your unique hair type and imbalances. Vata, Pitta, and Kapha are the three doshas or energy principles that govern our bodies, and each

dosha has specific characteristics that influence our hair. By identifying your dominant dosha, you can tailor your hair care routine accordingly.

For Vata hair, which tends to be dry and frizzy, regular oil massages using warm sesame or almond oil can help nourish and hydrate the scalp.

Pitta hair, which is prone to premature graying and thinning, benefits from cooling and calming oils like coconut or brahmi oil.

Kapha hair, on the other hand, tends to be oily and heavy, so light oils such as jojoba or mustard oilare recommended for balancing the scalp.

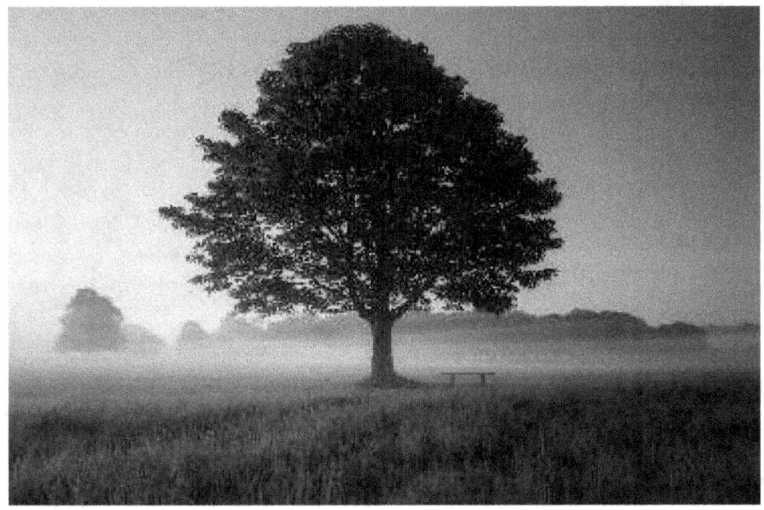

Besides oil massages, Ayurveda emphasizes the importance of a healthy diet for

maintaining lustrous hair.

Consuming foods rich in vitamins A, C, and E, such as leafy greens, citrus fruits, and nuts, can promote hair growth and strength. Additionally, incorporating Ayurvedic herbs like amla, bhringraj, and shikakai into your hair care routine can stimulate hair follicles and prevent hair loss.

Scalp treatments play a crucial role in Ayurvedic hair care as well. One popular

technique is Shirodhara, where a continuous stream of warm herbal oil is poured onto the forehead and scalp, inducing deep relaxation and nourishing the hair roots.

Another effective treatment is Nasya, which involves applying medicated oils or ghee to the

nostrils to cleanse and rejuvenate the scalp.

To maintain a healthy scalp, Ayurveda recommends avoiding harsh chemical-based hair products and opting for natural lternatives instead.

Gentle herbal shampoos, homemade hair masks using ingredients like yogurt and fenugreek, and natural hair rinses with herbal infusions can all promote scalp health and prevent common hair problems like dandruff and scalp irritation.

By incorporating Ayurvedic principles into your hair care routine, you can achieve not only beautiful and shiny hair but also a balanced and healthy scalp.

Remember, your hair reflects your overall health, and by nurturing it with natural Ayurvedic practices, you can enhance your beauty from within.

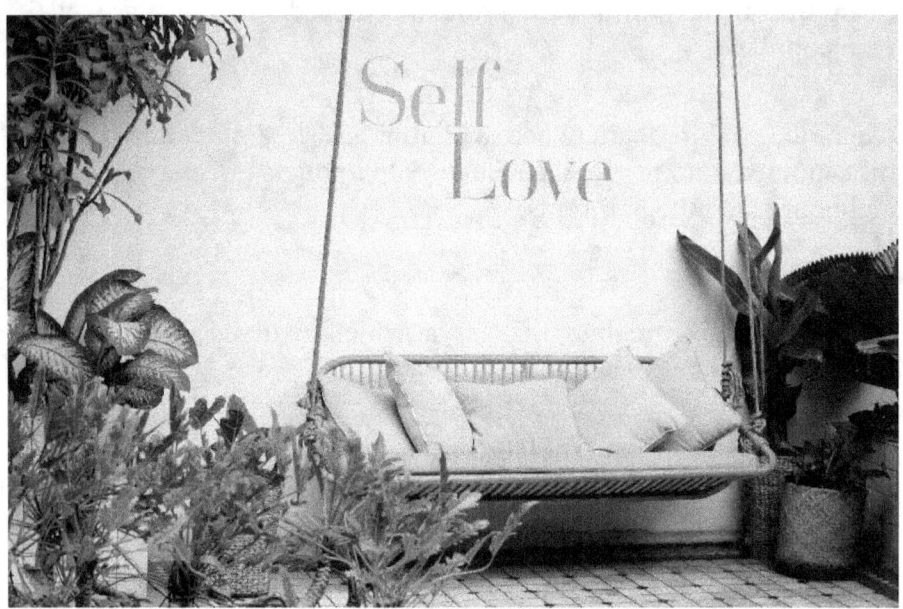

Ayurvedic Beauty Rituals for Radiant Skin and Hair

In today's fast-paced world, taking care of our health and beauty often falls by the wayside. However, Ayurveda offers timeless wisdom on how to enhance our health and beauty naturally.

Ayurvedic beauty rituals can help us achieve radiant skin and lustrous hair, while also promoting overall well- being. In this subchapter, we will explore some Ayurvedic practices that can transform your beauty regimen.

One of the key principles of Ayurveda is understanding your unique mind-body constitution, or dosha. By identifying your dominant dosha, you can tailor your beauty rituals to suit your individual needs.

For instance, if you are predominantly Pitta, with

fiery and sensitive skin, cooling and soothing ingredients like rose water and aloe vera can work wonders in calming your skin.

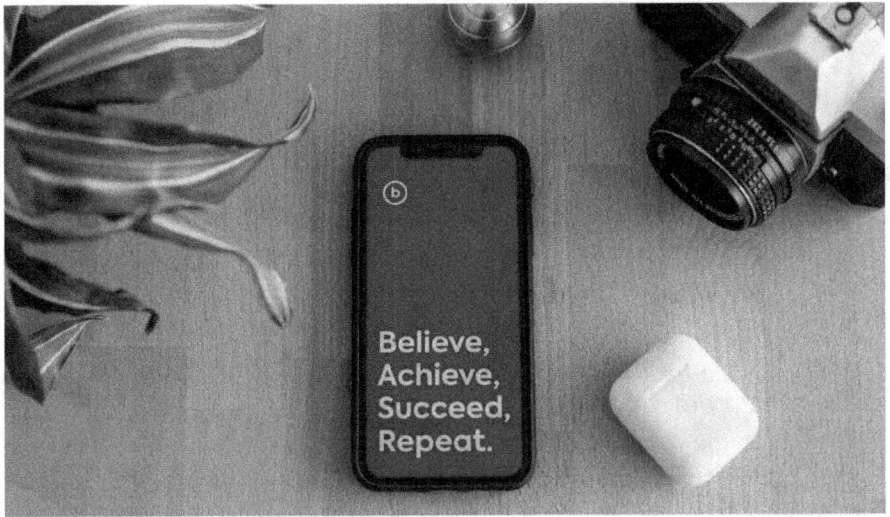

Cleansing is an essential step in any beauty routine, and Ayurveda emphasizes the use of natural ingredients to cleanse and purify the skin. A popular Ayurvedic practice is using

herbal powders or pastes, such as triphala or neem, to gently exfoliate and cleanse the

skin. These herbs possess powerful antibacterial and antifungal properties, promoting a clear and glowing complexion.

After cleansing, nourishing the skin becomes imperative. Ayurveda suggests using herbal oils, such as sesame or coconut oil, for daily self-massage, known as Abhyanga. This practice not only deeply moisturizes the skin but also improves blood circulation and promotes the removal of toxins. For those with oily skin, lighter oils like jojoba or almond oil can be used.

In addition to skincare, Ayurveda also offers valuable insights for maintaining healthy and lustrous hair. Regular scalp massages with warm herbal oils, such as Brahmi or Bhringraj, can stimulate hair growth, prevent dandruff, and nourish the scalp.

Ayurveda also recommends using natural hair cleansers like shikakai or reetha, which gently cleanse the hair without stripping it of its natural oils.

Lastly, Ayurveda emphasizes the importance of a balanced lifestyle and diet in promoting beauty from within. Consuming a variety of fresh fruits and vegetables, staying hydrated, and practicing stress management techniques like yoga and meditation can greatly enhance

your natural beauty.

In conclusion, Ayurvedic beauty rituals offer a holistic approach to enhancing your health and beauty naturally.

By understanding your dosha and incorporating Ayurvedic practices into your daily routine, you can achieve radiant skin and lustrous hair while also promoting overall well-being. Embrace the wisdom of Ayurveda and unlock the secrets to timeless beauty.

Furthermore, Ayurveda acknowledges the connection between diet and beauty.

It encourages a wholesome diet consisting of fresh, seasonal, and organic foods that are in line with your doshic constitution. By consuming nutritious meals and avoiding processed or artificial ingredients, you can enhance both your inner and outer beauty.

In conclusion, Ayurveda offers a comprehensive approach to health and beauty, focusing on balance, individuality, and self-care. By incorporating Ayurvedic principles and practices into your daily life, you can experience a profound transformation in your well-being

transformation in your well-being.

So, stay tuned, and get ready to embark on your journey towards vibrant

health and natural beauty with Ayurveda.

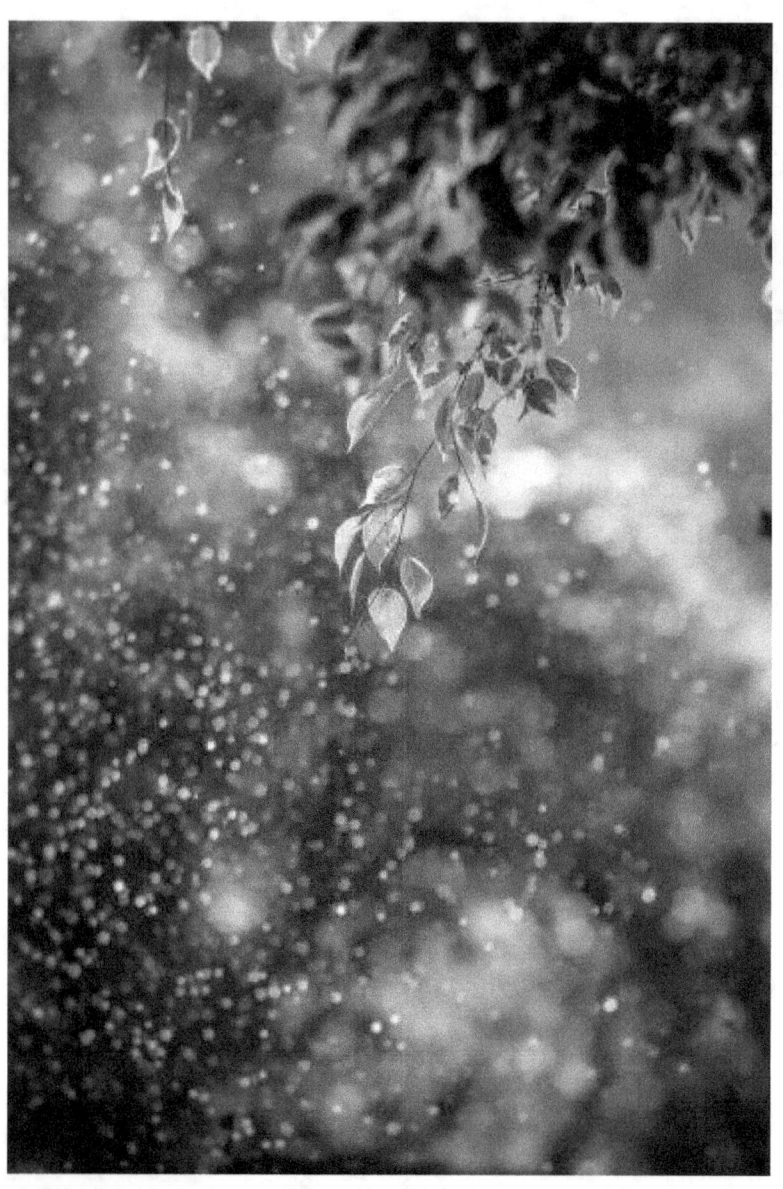

Introduction to Ayurvedic Herbs

Ayurveda, is an ancient Indian system of medicine, has gained popularity worldwide for its holistic approach to health and beauty.

Ayurvedic herbs play a vital role in this system, offering natural remedies to enhance not only our

physical well-being but also our inner radiance.

In this chapter, we will delve into the world of Ayurvedic herbs, exploring their benefits and how they can be incorporated into our daily lives.

Ayurvedic herbs are derived from various parts of plants, such as leaves, roots, bark, and seeds. These herbs are known for their therapeutic properties and have been used for centuries to treat ailments and promote overall wellness.

What sets Ayurvedic herbs apart is their ability to

restore balance to the body, mind, and spirit.

One of the fundamental concepts in Ayurveda is the belief that each person has a unique constitution known as doshas – Vata, Pitta, and Kapha. Ayurvedic herbs work in harmony with these doshas, helping to maintain their equilibrium and prevent diseases.

For example, Ashwagandha is a popular herb that helps reduce stress and anxiety, making it beneficial for individuals with an aggravated Vata dosha.

Ayurvedic herbs not only address physical ailments but also nourish our skin and

enhance our beauty.

Neem, known as the "divine tree," is a powerful herb that purifies the blood, preventing skin problems like acne and eczema.

Similarly, Turmeric, often referred to as the "golden spice," possesses antioxidant and anti-inflammatory properties, promoting a healthy complexion and slowing down the aging process.

Incorporating Ayurvedic herbs into your daily routine is easy. They can be consumed as herbal teas, supplements, or used topically in the form of oils, creams, or masks.

However, it is crucial to understand your unique constitution and consult an Ayurvedic practitioner to determine the most suitable herbs for your specific needs.

Throughout this book, we will explore a wide range of Ayurvedic herbs and their specific benefits, guiding you on how to integrate them into your health and beauty practices.

You will discover how to make herbal infusions, prepare homemade beauty remedies, and incorporate Ayurvedic herbs into your diet. By embracing these natural remedies, you can enhance your overall well-being and radiate beauty from within.

In the following chapters, we will delve deeper into the world of Ayurvedic herbs,

exploring their specific uses, dosha balancing properties, and effective applications.

Get ready to embark on a journey towards optimal health and natural beauty with the power of Ayurveda and its incredible herbs.

Common Ayurvedic Herbs for Health and Beauty

Ayurveda, the ancient Indian system of medicine, offers a wealth of knowledge about natural remedies for enhancing health and beauty.

In this chapter, we will explore some of the most commonly used

Ayurvedic herbs that can help you achieve a healthy and radiant appearance.

1. Aloe Vera: Known for its soothing and healing properties, aloe vera is a versatile herb

that can be used both externally and internally. It helps to nourish the skin, promote hair growth, and improve digestion, making it an essential herb for overall health and beauty.

2. Turmerc: Considered the "queen of spices," turmeric has powerful anti-inflammatory and antioxidant properties. It helps to improve the complexion, reduce acne, and promote a natural glow. Turmeric can be used in face masks, body scrubs, and even consumed in dishes to reap its numerous benefits.

3. Neem: Neem is a popular herb known for its antibacterial

and antifungal properties. It helps to treat acne, reduce inflammation, and cleanse the skin. Neem can be used in the form of oil, powder, or as an ingredient in skincare products to achieve clear and healthy skin.

4. Brahmi: This herb is often referred to as the "memory enhancer" as it helps improve cognitive function and memory. Brahmi also nourishes the scalp, promotes hair growth, and

prevents premature greying. It can be consumed as a supplement or used in hair oils to reap its benefits.

5. Ashwagandha: Known as anadaptogenic herb, ashwagandha helps the body cope with stress and promotes overall wellness. It also has anti-aging properties and can help reduce wrinkles, improve skin elasticity, and promote a youthful appearance.

6. Triphala: This powerful herbal blend consists of three fruits - Amalaki, Bibhitaki, and Haritaki. Triphala helps to cleanse and detoxify the body, improve digestion, and enhance the absorption of nutrients. It is often used as a daily supplement for overall health and vitality.

These are just a few examples of commonly used Ayurvedic herbs for health and beauty.

Incorporating these herbs into your daily routine can help you achieve a natural and holistic approach to wellness.

However, it is essential to consult a qualified Ayurvedic practitioner before introducing any new herbs or supplements into your routine, as everyone's body is unique and may react differently to certain herbs.

With the guidance of an expert, you can harness the power of Ayurveda to enhance your health and beauty naturally.

Preparing and Using Ayurvedic Herbal Remedies

Ayurveda, the ancient Indian system of medicine, offers a holistic approach to health and beauty. One of its key

principles is the use of herbal remedies to address various ailments and enhance overall well-being. In this subchapter, we will delve into the world of Ayurvedic

herbal remedies, exploring how to prepare and use them effectively.

When it comes to preparing Ayurvedic herbal remedies, it is crucial to emphasize the use of high-quality, organic herbs. This ensures that the remedies are free from harmful chemicals and additives, promoting optimal health benefits.

It is recommended to source herbs from reputable suppliers or consider growing your own herbal garden.

To prepare Ayurvedic herbal remedies, there are several methods you can explore. One popular method is making herbal infusions or teas. This involves steeping herbs in hot water to extract their medicinal properties. An important aspect of this process is determining the appropriate dosage and duration of steeping to maximize the potency of the remedy.

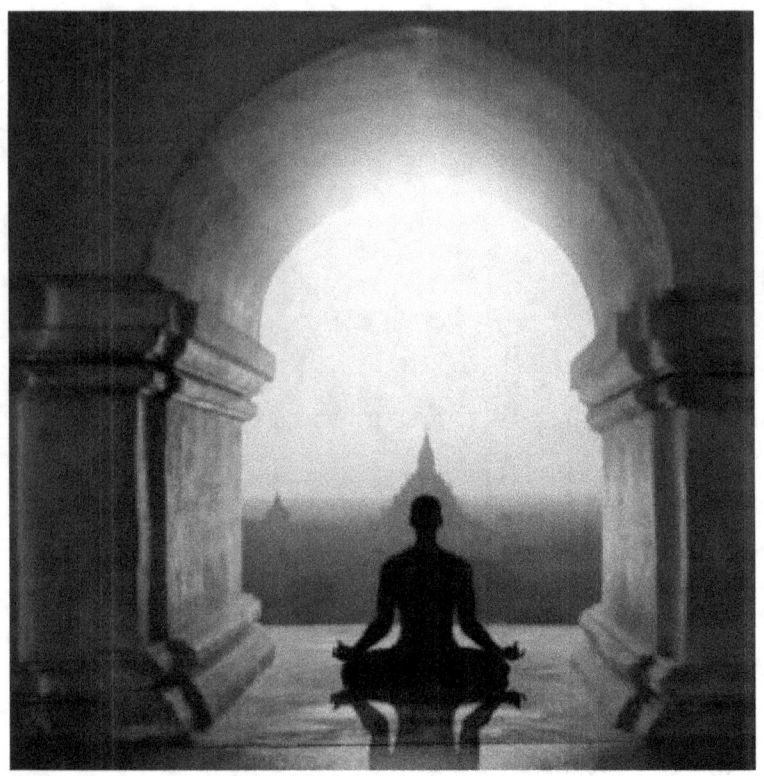

Another method is creating herbal

decoctions, which involve boiling herbs in water until the liquid reduces to a

concentrated form. Decoctions are particularly useful for extracting the medicinal properties of hard or woody herbs.

I
t is crucial to follow precise

instructions and measurements to ensure the desired concentration is achieved.

In addition to teas and decoctions,

Ayurveda also utilizes herbal powders and pastes. These can be mixed with various carriers such as honey or ghee to create potent remedies. It is important to note

that the dosage and application of these remedies should be based on individual

needs and constitution, as recommended by an Ayurvedic practitioner.

When using Ayurvedic herbal remedies, it is essential to be mindful of any

potential allergies or contraindications. It is advisable to consult with an Ayurvedic expert or healthcare professional before incorporating any new remedies into

your routine, especially if you have pre- existing medical conditions or are taking medications.

In conclusion, Ayurvedic herbal remedies offer a natural and holistic approach to health and beauty.

By understanding the methods of preparation and usage, you can harness the full potential of these remedies to

enhance your well-being.

Remember to prioritize the use of high-quality herbs and seek professional guidance when needed.

So, embark on a journey towards optimal health and beauty, naturally.

Herbal Remedies for Common Ailments

In the world of Ayurveda, the ancient Indian system of medicine, herbal remedies have been used for centuries to treat common ailments and promote overall health and

beauty. These natural remedies offer a gentle and holistic approach to healing, focusing on the body as a whole rather than just the symptoms.

One of the most common ailments that can be effectively treated with herbal remedies is the common cold. Instead of reaching for over-the-counter medications, Ayurveda

recommends using herbs such as ginger, turmeric, and basil to boost the immune

system and alleviate symptoms. Ginger tea with a dash of turmeric and a few leaves of basil can provide relief from congestion, cough, and sore throat.

Another common issue that can be addressed with herbal remedies is digestive problems.

Ayurveda believes that a healthy digestive system is key to overall well-bloating, fennel seeds and peppermint being. For those suffering from indigestion or tea can work wonders. Fennel seeds can be chewed after a meal to aid digestion, while peppermint tea helps soothe the stomach and relieve discomfort.

When it comes to skincare, Ayurveda offers a plethora of herbal remedies for various skin conditions. For acne-prone skin, neem, turmeric, and sandalwood are highly recommended. Neem has antibacterial properties that can help fight acne-causing bacteria, while turmeric acts as an anti-inflammatory agent and sandalwood has a cooling effect on the skin.

A paste made from these herbs can be applied as a face mask to reduce inflammation and promote clear and healthy skin.

Hair loss is another concern that can be effectively tackled with Ayurvedic herbal remedies. Amla, also known as Indian gooseberry, is a potent herb that strengthens hair follicles and promotes hair growth. Amla oil can be massaged into the scalp to nourish the hair roots and prevent hair fall.

Overall, Ayurvedic herbal remedies offer a natural and holistic approach to common ailments and beauty concerns. These remedies have stood the test of time and are trusted by

millions around the world.

By incorporating these practices into your daily routine, you can enhance your health and beauty naturally, without the need for harsh chemicals or

medications.

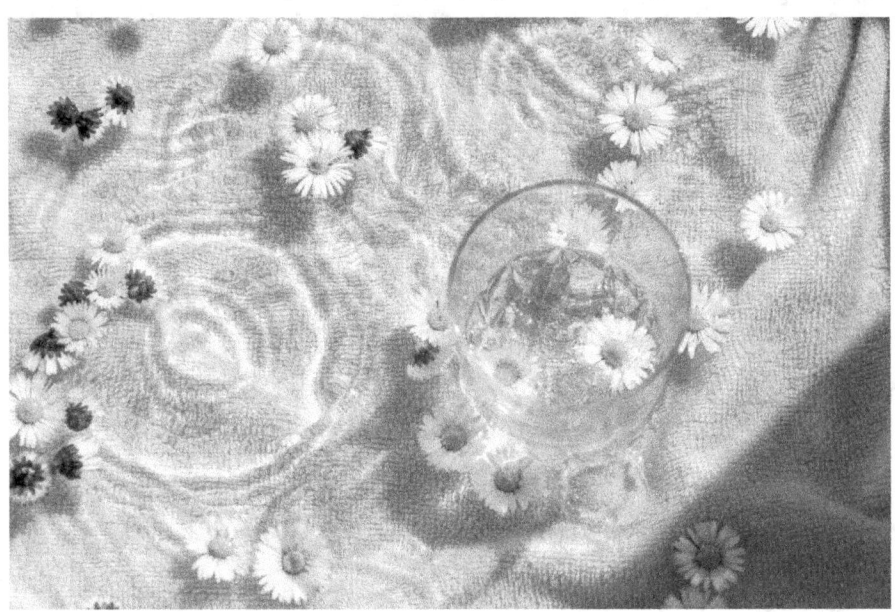

Ayurvedic Herbal Supplements and Formulations

In the realm of Ayurveda, herbal supplements and formulations play a vital role in promoting overall health and beauty naturally.

Ayurvedic practitioners have been utilizing the power of herbs for centuries to enhance physical and mental well-being. These herbal supplements are derived from various parts of plants, including leaves, roots, stems, and fruits, and are known for their therapeutic properties.

One of the key principles in Ayurveda is the belief that every individual possesses a unique constitution or dosha, namely Vata, Pitta, or Kapha. Herbal supplements and formulations are tailored to balance and harmonize these doshas, promoting optimal health and beauty. These natural remedies help address specific health concerns, boost the immune system, and rejuvenate the body and mind.

Ayurvedic herbal supplements are available in various forms, such as powders, tablets, capsules, and oils. They are created by combining different herbs, known as formulations, to enhance their efficacy.

These formulations are carefully crafted to support specific health needs, such as improving digestion, boosting energy levels, strengthening the immune system, or promoting radiant skin and lustrous hair.

Some popular Ayurvedic herbal supplements include Triphala, Ashwagandha, Brahmi, Tulsi, and Turmeric. Triphala, a combination of three fruits, is renowned for its detoxifying and digestive properties. Ashwagandha, also known as Indian ginseng, is a powerful adaptogen that helps reduce stress and promotes overall vitality.

Brahmi enhances cognitive functions, memory, and concentration, while Tulsi acts as a natural immune booster. Turmeric, with its potent anti-inflammatory properties, is widely used for both internal consumption and topical application.

It is essential to consult an Ayurvedic practitioner or a qualified health care professional before incorporating herbal supplements into your routine. They can provide personalized guidance based on your dosha and specific health needs. It is important to remember that Ayurvedic herbal supplements work synergistically with other Ayurvedic health and beauty practices, such as diet, lifestyle modifications, and holistic therapies.

By incorporating Ayurvedic herbal supplements and formulations into your daily routine, you can tap into the immense healing potential of nature.

These natural remedies can help restore balance, promote vitality, and enhance your overall well-being. Embrace the wisdom of Ayurveda and experience the transformative power of herbal supplements for a healthier and more beautiful you.

Ayurvedic Approach to Stress and Anxiety

In today's fast-paced world, stress and anxiety have become all too common. We find ourselves constantly juggling work, family, and personal obligations, leaving little time for self-care and

relaxation. Fortunately, Ayurveda, the ancient Indian system of medicine,

Fortunately, Ayurveda, the ancient Indian system of medicine, offers a holistic approach to managing stress and anxiety, promoting overall well-being and balance.

Ayurveda views stress and anxiety as imbalances in the mind and body, caused by various factors such as lifestyle choices, diet, and environmental influences.

According to Ayurveda, each individual has a unique constitution, known as doshas Vata, Pitta, and Kapha), and imbalances in these doshas can contribute to stress and anxiety.

One of the key principles of Ayurveda is maintaining a healthy lifestyle, which includes following a regular routine and adopting practices that promote relaxation and rejuvenation. These practices can help calm the mind, reduce stress, and restore balance in the body.

Ayurveda recommends stress-reducing herbs and spices into your daily routine.

your daily routine. Ashwagandha, Brahmi, and Tulsi are well-known Ayurvedic herbs that have adaptogenic properties, helping the body adapt to stress and promoting a sense of calm.

Another important aspect of Ayurveda is the practice of self-care rituals, known as Dinacharya. This involves establishing a daily routine that includes activities such as oil massage Abhyanga), meditation, and yoga. Abhyanga, or self-massage, helps nourish the body, relax the muscles, and calm the mind. Meditation and yoga, on the other hand, help release tension, improve focus, and promote a sense of inner peace.

Ayurvedic dietary guidelines also play a crucial role in managing stress and anxiety. Consuming a balanced diet that includes whole grains, fresh fruits and vegetables, and healthy fats can provide the body with essential nutrients and support overall well-being.

well-being.

Avoiding processed foods, caffeine, and excessive sugar can help prevent energy crashes and promote a stable mood.

By incorporating Ayurvedic practices such as self-care rituals, herbal supplements, and a balanced diet into your daily routine, you can enhance your overall health and beauty naturally.

Digestive Disorders and Ayurvedic Solutions

In today's fast-paced world, digestive disorders have become increasingly

common. From indigestion and bloating to more serious conditions like irritable bowel syndrome and acid reflux, these issues can greatly impact our overall well-being.

Fortunately, Ayurveda offers a holistic approach to tackle these digestive disorders and restore balance these digestive disorders and restore balance to our bodies digestive system.

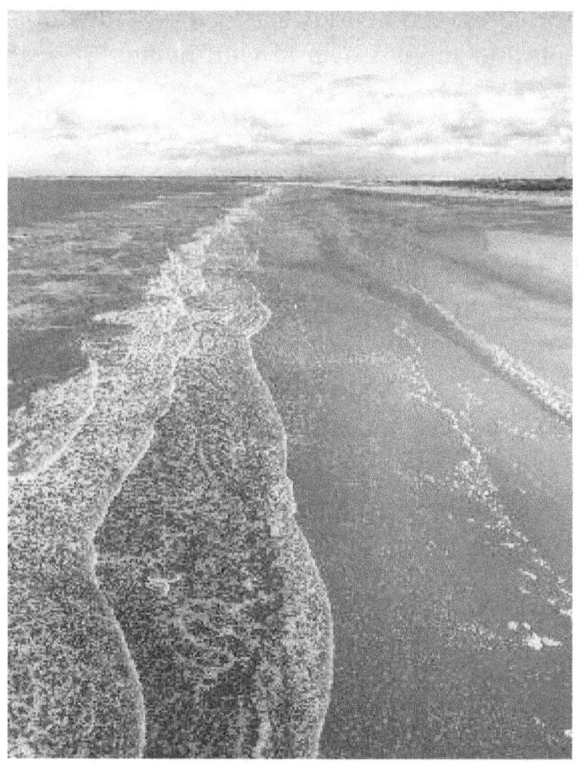

Ayurveda, the ancient Indian science of healing and wellness, emphasizes the importance of maintaining a healthy

According to Ayurveda, a well-functioning digestive system is the cornerstone of good health. When our digestion is compromised, it can lead to a variety of issues that affect not only our physical well-being but also our beauty.

One of the key principles of Ayurveda is the concept of 'agni,' which refers to the digestive fire. This fire is responsible for breaking down the food we consume

and extracting the nutrients our bodies need.

When our agni is weak or imbalanced, it can result in poor digestion, leading to various digestive disorders.

To address these issues, Ayurveda

offers a range of natural solutions that target the root causes of digestive

disorders. These solutions include dietary changes, herbal remedies, lifestyle modifications, and specific practices to strengthen the digestive system.

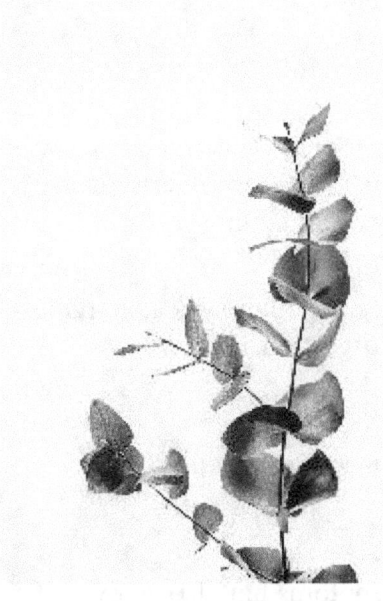

A balanced Ayurvedic diet plays a vital role in maintaining optimal digestion. It emphasizes the consumption of easily digestible foods, such as cooked vegetables, whole grains, and herbal teas.

Additionally, Ayurveda recommends avoiding processed

foods, excessive consumption of cold or raw foods, and incompatible food combinations, which can hinder digestion.

Herbal remedies are another integral part of Ayurvedic solutions for digestive disorders.

Ayurveda offers a plethora of herbs and spices that can aid digestion, reduce

inflammation, and soothe the digestive tract. Common herbs used in Ayurvedic remedies include ginger, fennel, turmeric, and peppermint.

In addition to dietary and herbal interventions, Ayurveda emphasizes the importance of lifestyle modifications to support digestive health. These include practicing mindful eating, maintaining

a regular eating schedule, and engaging in gentle physical activities like yoga or walking after meals to aid digestion.

By implementing Ayurvedic solutions for digestive disorders, individuals can

experience not only relief from their symptoms but also an overall improvement in their health and beauty.

Ayurveda's holistic approach recognizes the interconnectedness of the body, mind, and spirit, and aims to restore balance in all aspects of our being.

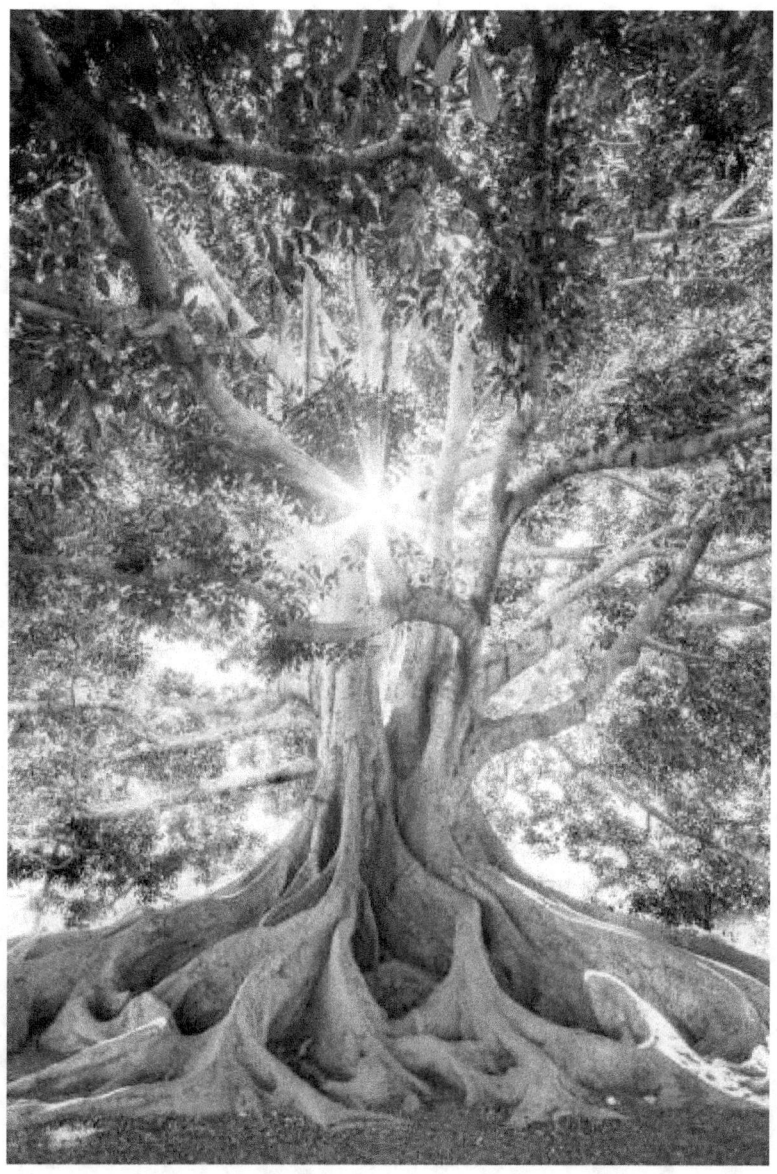

In conclusion, Ayurveda offers a comprehensive approach to address digestive

disorders. Its emphasis on nutrition, herbal remedies, and lifestyle modifications can help individuals achieve optimal digestive health and enhance their overall well-being naturally.

Ayurvedic Remedies for Skin Conditions

In the world of Ayurveda, achieving optimal health and beauty is not only about external self-care but also internal balance. Ayurvedic remedies for skin conditions focus on

restoring harmony within the body, promoting healthy and glowing skin naturally.

Let's explore some ancient Ayurvedic practices that can help you achieve clear and radiant skin.

One of the most fundamental principles of Ayurveda is understanding the unique constitution of each individual, known as doshas – Vata, Pitta, and Kapha. Skin

conditions often arise due to an imbalance in these doshas, and Ayurveda offers personalized remedies for each dosha type.

For Vata skin, which tends to be dry and prone to fine lines and wrinkles, nourishment and hydration are key.

Incorporating warm sesame oil massages, both internally and externally, can deeply moisturize the skin and improve its elasticity. Additionally, using natural remedies like rose water, aloe vera, and almond oil can help soothe and hydrate Vata skin.

Pitta skin, on the other hand, is more prone to inflammation, acne, and sensitivity. To pacify Pitta dosha, Ayurveda recommends cooling and calming remedies.

Applying a paste of sandalwood, turmeric, and rose water can help reduce redness and soothe irritated skin. Consuming cooling foods like cucumber, coconut water, and cilantro can also help balance Pitta from within.

Kapha skin is typically oily and prone to congestion and acne. Ayurvedic remedies for Kapha skin focus on detoxification and balancing excess oil.

Regular exfoliation with natural ingredients like chickpea flour, turmeric, and honey can help reduce oiliness and unclog pores. Incorporating herbs like neem and tea tree oil into skincare routines can also help combat acne and purify the skin.

Apart from dosha-specific remedies, Ayurveda emphasizes a holistic approach to skincare. Practices like abhyanga (self-massage), yoga, and meditation can promote overall well-

being, reducing stress and promoting healthy skin. Ayurveda also emphasizes the

importance of a balanced diet, incorporating fresh fruits, vegetables, and herbs to nourish the skin from within.

Remember, Ayurvedic remedies for skin conditions work best when combined with a

healthy lifestyle and a customized approach based on your dosha type. Consultation with an Ayurvedic practitioner can provide deeper insights into your unique constitution and guide you towards a personalized skincare routine.

Women's Health and Ayurveda

Ayurveda, the ancient Indian system of medicine, offers a holistic approach to women's health and well-being. With its emphasis on natural remedies and a balanced lifestyle, Ayurveda provides women with powerful tools to enhance their health and beauty naturally. In this subchapter, we will explore the various Ayurvedic health and beauty practices specifically tailored for women.

One of the key principles of Ayurveda is understanding the unique constitution of each individual. Women are no exception, as their bodies undergo various physiological changes throughout their lives.

importance of hormonal balance and

offers specific herbs and treatments to support women's reproductive health.

From menstrual irregularities to

menopause, Ayurveda provides natural

solutions to alleviate common symptoms and restore balance.

Ayurvedic nutrition plays a vital role in women's health. The right diet can help restore hormonal balance, improve digestion, and boost energy levels. Ayurveda recommends foods that are nourishing and supportive for women, such as whole grains, fresh fruits and vegetables, and healthy fats. Additionally, specific herbs and spices are known for their therapeutic properties in addressing women's health concerns. For instance,

For instance, shatavari is highly regarded for its ability to regulate hormonal imbalances, while turmeric is known for its anti-inflammatory properties.

In addition to diet and herbal remedies, Ayurveda emphasizes the importance of self- care practices for women.

Abhyanga, the practice of self-massage with warm oils, not only nourishes the skin but also helps balance the body and mind.

Regular exercise, such as yoga and walking, is also recommended to maintain overall health and vitality.

Ayurveda also encourages women to cultivate a daily routine that includes adequate sleep, stress management techniques, and mindfulness practices.

Furthermore, Ayurveda recognizes the importance of mental and emotional well-being for women. Stress, anxiety, and emotional imbalances can have a significant impact on women's health. Ayurvedic practices such as meditation, deep breathing exercises, and specific herbal formulations can help support women's emotional balance and promote overall mental well-being.

In conclusion, Ayurveda offers a comprehensive approach to women's health and

beauty. By understanding and addressing individual needs, following a balanced diet,

engaging in self-care practices, and nurturing mental and emotional well-being, women can enhance their overall health and vitality naturally.

By incorporating Ayurvedic principles into their lives, women can achieve a harmonious balance between their bodies, minds, and spirits, leading to lasting health and beauty.

Ayurveda for Weight Management

In today's fast-paced world, weight management has become a significant concern for many individuals. People are constantly searching for effective and natural ways to shed those extra pounds and achieve a healthier body. Ayurveda, the ancient Indian system of medicine, offers

a holistic approach to weight management that focuses on balancing the mind, body, and spirit.

Ayurveda views weight gain as a result of an imbalance in the body's doshas or energy forces.

According to this system, there are three primary doshas: Vata, Pitta, and Kapha. Each dosha

governs specific functions in the body, and an imbalance in any of these doshas can lead to weight gain.

To address weight management through Ayurveda, it is crucial to identify your dominant

dosha understand how it affects your body.

For instance, individuals with excess Vata energy may experience weight gain due to irregular eating habits and stress.

Pitta-dominant individuals may struggle with weight gain due to poor digestion and an imbalanced metabolism.

Kapha-dominant individuals tend to have a slower metabolism and may gain weight easily.

Ayurveda offers various natural remedies and practices to help balance the doshas and manage weight effectively. These practices include dietary changes, lifestyle modifications, herbal treatments, and regular exercise.

In terms of diet, Ayurveda emphasizes the importance of eating whole, unprocessed foods that are suitable for your dosha. It recommends incorporating spices like turmeric, ginger, and cumin into your meals to aid digestion and boost metabolism.

Additionally, practicing mindful eating, such as chewing food thoroughly and eating in a calm environment, can also contribute to weight management.

Ayurveda also highlights the significance of a balanced lifestyle to maintain a healthy weight. This includes getting enough sleep, managing stress through practices like meditation and yoga, and engaging in regular physical activity.

Exercise is essential, but it should be tailored to your dosha. Vata-dominant individuals may benefit from gentle activities like walking or yoga, while Pitta and Kapha types may benefit from more intense exercises.

Furthermore, Ayurveda utilizes various herbal remedies to support weight

management. Herbs like triphala, guggulu, and ginger can aid digestion, boost

metabolism, and reduce cravings. However, it is crucial to consult an

Ayurvedic practitioner before incorporating any herbal supplements into your routine.

In conclusion, Ayurveda provides a comprehensive and natural approach to weight managemen. By understanding your dosha and making appropriate changes to your diet and ncorporating,

herbal remedies in your lifestyle, you can achieve a healthier and more balanced body.

Remember, it is always best to consult an Ayurvedic practitioner to tailor a weight program.

Ayurvedic Practices for Longevity

In the quest for health and beauty, many people are turning to ancient practices that have withstood the test of time. One such practice is Ayurveda, a holistic system of medicine that originated in India thousands of years ago. Ayurveda not only focuses on treating diseases but also emphasizes preventive measures to promote longevity and overall well-being.

Ayurveda recognizes that each person is unique and has a distinct constitution or dosha. There are three primary doshas: Vata, Pitta, and Kapha. Understanding yourdosha can help you make informed choices about diet, lifestyle, and herbal remedies to maintain balance and promote longevity.

One of the fundamental principles of Ayurveda for longevity is maintaining a healthy digestive system. According to Ayurveda, a strong digestive fire, or "agni," is crucial for optimal health. To enhance agni, Ayurveda recommends consuming warm, freshly prepared meals that are easy to digest.

Avoiding processed foods, excessive snacking, and overeating can also support a robust digestive system.

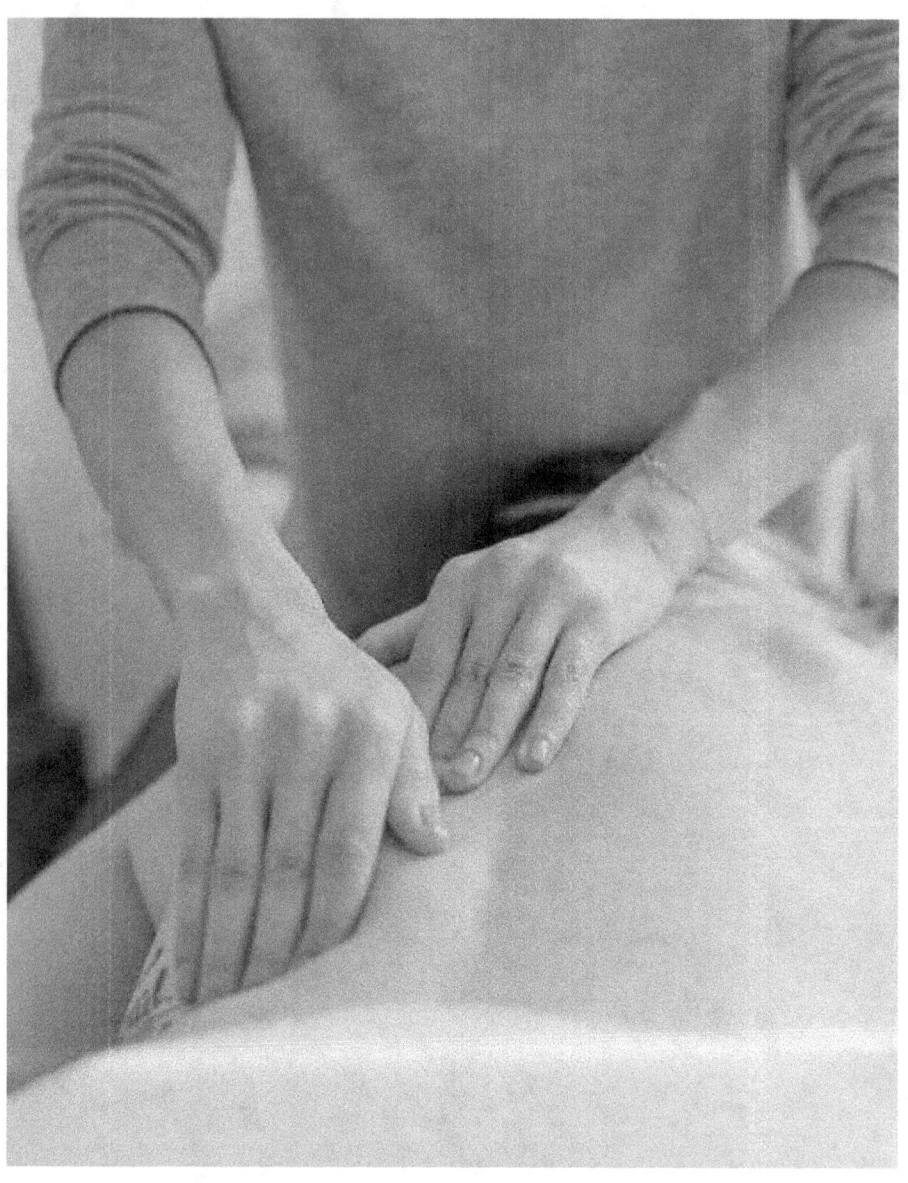

In addition to a balanced diet, Ayurveda suggests incorporating specific herbs and spices

into your daily routine to promote longevity. For example, turmeric, a potent antioxidant and anti-inflammatory herb, is known for its ability to boost immunity and support healthy aging. Ashwagandha, another powerful herb, is known for its adaptogenic properties, helping the body cope with stress and promoting longevity.

Ayurvedic practices for longevity also include daily self-care rituals, known as "dinacharya."

These rituals may involve tongue scraping, oil pulling, and self-massage with herbal oils.

Tongue scraping helps remove toxins and promotes oral hygiene, while oil pulling detoxifies the mouth and supports overall oral health.

Self-massage, or "abhyanga," with warm herbal oils nourishes the skin, improves blood circulation, and promotes relaxation.

Furthermore, Ayurveda emphasizes the importance of maintaining a healthy sleep routine. Getting adequate restful sleep is vital for the body's rejuvenation and overall longevity.

Ayurveda recommends going to bed early, avoiding stimulating activities before sleep, and creating a peaceful sleep environment to support a deep and restorative slumber.

In conclusion, Ayurvedic practices for longevity offer a holistic approach to health and beauty. By understanding your unique constitution, nurturing your digestive system,

incorporating specific herbs and spices, and embracing self-care rituals and healthy sleep habits, you can enhance your overall well-being and promote longevity naturally.

Embracing these Ayurvedic principles can help you lead a balanced and fulfilling life while unlocking the secrets to a youthful and radiant appearance.

Ayurvedic Anti-Aging Techniques

In our modern world, where stress and pollution are rampant, it has become

increasingly important to seek natural and holistic approaches to maintaining our

health and beauty.

Ayurveda, the ancient Indian healing system, offers a wealth of knowledge and techniques to help us combat the signs of aging and enhance our overall well-being.

Ayurvedic anti-aging techniques focus on promoting balance and harmony within

the body, mind, and spirit. By addressing the root causes of aging, rather than

merely treating the symptoms, Ayurveda provides a comprehensive approach to

slowing down the aging process naturally.

One of the key principles of Ayurveda is the concept of doshas, which are the

unique energies that govern our physical and mental characteristics. Understanding your dosha type can help you tailor your anti-aging practices to suit your individual needs.

To maintain a youthful appearance, Ayurveda emphasizes the importance of proper nutrition. Consuming a balanced diet that includes fresh fruits, vegetables, whole grains, and lean proteins nourishes the body from within and supports healthy aging. Specific herbs, such as ashwagandha and turmeric, are also recommended for their rejuvenating properties.

importance of detoxification to remove harmful toxins from the body. Regular detoxification practices, such as herbal cleanses and oil massages, help to purify the system and enhance the body's natural ability to regenerate and repair itself.

In addition to internal practices, Ayurveda offers a range of external treatments to promote youthful skin and overall beauty. Facial massages with Ayurvedic oils,

known as Abhyanga, not only relax the mind but also stimulate blood circulation and encourage the removal of toxins.

The use of natural herbal face masks and scrubs can further enhance the skin's

glow and reduce the appearance of wrinkles and fine lines.

Ayurvedic anti-aging techniques also emphasize the importance of stress management. Chronic stress canaccelerate the aging process, leading to premature wrinkles and other signs of aging.

Ayurveda recommends practices such as meditation, yoga, and breathing exercises to calm the mind and reduce stress levels, promoting a youthful and radiant appearance.

By incorporating Ayurvedic anti-aging techniques into your daily routine, you can

enhance your health and beauty naturally.

Embracing the holistic principles of Ayurveda and making conscious choices to support your well-being will not only slow down the aging process but also bring about a sense of balance and harmony in your life. Remember, true beauty radiates from within, and Ayurveda offers a pathway to unlock your natural glow and vitality. Start your journey towards timeless beauty today by embracing the wisdom of Ayurvedic anti-aging techniques.

Ayurvedic Herbs and Formulations for Anti-Aging

In our quest for eternal youth and beauty, many of us turn to expensive creams,

serums, and procedures.

However, Ayurveda, the ancient Indian system of medicine, provides us with a treasure trove of natural remedies for anti-aging. Ayurvedic

herbs and formulations have been used for centuries to enhance health and beauty naturally, and their effectiveness is being recognized by people around the world.

In this chapter, we will explore some of the most potent Ayurvedic herbs and formulations that can help you slow down the aging process and maintain a youthful glow.

One of the key principles of Ayurveda is the belief that beauty and aging are deeply

connected to the balance of the doshas, or energy forces, within our body. Imbalances in the doshas can lead to premature aging and various health issues.

Ayurvedic herbs such as Ashwagandha, Amalaki, and Shatavari work to balance the doshas, promoting overall well-being and combating the signs of aging.

Ashwagandha, also known as Indian ginseng, is a powerful adaptogen that helps the

body adapt to stress and boosts energy levels. It is rich in antioxidants that protect the

skin from free radicals and reduce the appearance of wrinkles and fine lines.

Amalaki, or Indian gooseberry, is a potent source of vitamin C and other antioxidants, which help to rejuvenate the skin, promote collagen production, and improve skin elasticity.

Shatavari, known as the "queen of herbs," has anti-inflammatory properties and helps to nourish and hydrate the skin, reducing the appearance of dryness and wrinkles.

In addition to these individual herbs,

Ayurveda also offers a range of

formulations that combine multiple

herbs to target specific signs of aging.

Chyawanprash, a traditional Ayurvedic jam, is a blend of over 40 herbs and is renowned for its anti-aging properties. It boosts immunity, improves digestion, and promotes cellular regeneration, resulting in radiant and youthful skin.

Triphala, another popular Ayurvedic formulation, is a combination of three

fruits – Amalaki, Bibhitaki, and Haritaki. It detoxifies the body, enhances

digestion, and supports healthy aging.

Incorporating Ayurvedic herbs and formulations into your daily routine can have a profound impact on your health and beauty. However, it is important to consult an Ayurvedic practitioner or a qualified healthcare professional before starting any new herbal regimen.

They can provide personalized guidance based on your unique constitution and health needs. By harnessing the power of Ayurveda, you can enhance your health and beauty naturally, and

embrace the process of aging with grace and vitality.

Ayurvedic Practices for Maintaining Youthful Skin

In a world filled with countless beauty

products and skincare routines, it is easy to get overwhelmed.

However, Ayurveda, the ancient Indian

system of medicine, offers a holistic approach to health and beauty. Ayurvedic practices focus on restoring balance within the body, mind, and spirit, resulting in natural and long- lasting beauty.

In this chapter, we will explore Ayurvedic practices specifically tailored to maintain youthful skin.

Understanding Ayurvedic Principles:

According to Ayurveda, each individual possesses a unique combination of three doshas: Vata, Pitta, and Kapha. These doshas determine our physical and mental characteristics. Understanding your dominant dosha can help you choose the most suitable skincare regimen.

Ayurvedic Skincare Regimen:

1. Cleansing: Begin your skincare routine with a gentle cleanser that suits your dosha. Use natural ingredients like neem, rose water, or sandalwood to cleanse and purify the skin.

2. Exfoliation: Regular exfoliation removes dead skin cells and promotes cell turnover. Use natural exfoliants like oatmeal, rice flour, or finely ground herbs mixed with water or rose water to gently scrub your face.

3. Moisturization: Apply natural moisturizers like almond oil, coconut oil, or aloe vera gel to nourish and hydrate your skin.

Choose ingredients that suit your dosha and leave your skin feeling supple.

4. Facial Massage: A daily facial massage with herbal oils increases blood circulation and promotes lymphatic drainage. This helps nourish the skin, reduce wrinkles, and improve skin elasticity.

5. Herbal Masks: Applying homemade herbal masks can rejuvenate the skin. Use ingredients like turmeric, honey, yogurt, and sandalwood powder to create a mask that suits your dosha and addresses specific skin concerns.

6. Dietary Considerations: A healthy diet is crucial for maintaining youthful skin. Consume fresh fruits, vegetables, whole grains, and drink plenty of water. Avoid

excessive spicy, oily, or processed foods

that can aggravate your dosha.

7. Lifestyle Habits: Get enough sleep, manage stress, and practice regular exercise to maintain overall health and vibrant skin. Avoid smoking and limit alcohol consumption as they can accelerate skin aging.

Conclusion:

Ayurveda offers a comprehensive approach to maintaining youthful skin by considering an individual's unique dosha and promoting inner balance.

By following a tailored skincare regimen, incorporating natural ingredients, and making mindful lifestyle choices, you can enhance your health and beauty naturally.

Embrace the wisdom of Ayurveda, and let your skin radiate with youthful glow and vitality.

Mind-Body Practices for Aging Gracefully

In today's fast-paced world, with stress and pollution taking a toll on our health, it has become increasingly important to adopt holistic approaches to maintain our well-being.

Ayurveda, the ancient Indian system of medicine, offers a treasure trove of wisdom and practices that can enhance our health and beauty naturally.

One of the key aspects of Ayurveda is the mind-body connection, which acknowledges that our mental state directly affects our physical well-being. In this subchapter, we will explore some mind-body practices that can help us age gracefully.

These practices include:

1. Meditation: Meditation is a powerful technique that allows us to calm the mind, reduce stress, and promote inner peace.

Regular meditation practice has been scientifically proven to lower blood pressure, improve sleep quality, and reduce anxiety and depression. By incorporating meditation into

our daily routine, we can cultivate a sense of tranquility and emotional well-being, which reflects in our physical appearance.

2. Yoga: Yoga is a holistic practice that combines physical postures, breathing exercises, and meditation. Regular yoga practice helps improve flexibility, strength, and balance, while also promoting mental clarity and emotional stability. Certain yoga posters, such as the

shoulder stand or legs- up-the-wall pose, are specifically beneficial for slowing down

the aging process, as they enhance blood circulation to the face and scalp.

scalp.

3. Pranayama: Pranayama refers to various breathing exercises that can help balance the energy in our bodies. Deep breathing exercises, such as alternate nostril breathing or belly breathing, help increase oxygen supply to the cells, improve digestion, and boost overall vitality

By practicing pranayama regularly, we can enhance our energy levels, reduce stress, and promote a youthful glow.

4.Mindful Eating: Ayurveda emphasizes the importance of mindful eating, which involves being fully present and aware of the food we consume. By savoring each bite, chewing slowly, and paying attention to our body's hunger and fullness cues, we can improve digestion, prevent overeating, and promote better nutrient absorption. Eating a balanced, nourishing diet that includes fresh fruits, vegetables, whole grains, and healthy fats is essential for maintaining youthful vitality.

By incorporating these mind-body practices into our daily lives, we can enhance our health and beauty naturally.

Ayurveda teaches us that true beauty radiates from within and is a reflection of our overall well-being. So, let's embrace these practices and embark on a journey towards aging gracefully, with a healthy body, a calm mind, and a radiant spirit.

Creating a Personalized Ayurvedic Routine

Ayurveda, an ancient system of medicine and wellness, offers a holistic approach to health and beauty.

By understanding our unique mind-body constitution, known as doshas, we can create a personalized Ayurvedic routine that enhances our overall well-being.

This chapter will guide you through the process of discovering your dosha and incorporating Ayurvedic health and beauty practices into your daily life. Understanding Your Dosha.

In Ayurveda, there are three doshas: Vata, Pitta, and Kapha. Each dosha has specific characteristics that influence our physical, mental, and emotional well-being. By

identifying your dominant dosha, you can tailor your Ayurvedic routine to address your specific needs.

To determine your dosha, consider both your physical and mental attributes.

Are you prone to dry skin and hair?

Do you have a fiery temperament or a calm disposition?

Ayurvedic quizzes and consultations with Ayurvedic practitioners can help you identify your dosha with more accuracy.

Designing Your Ayurvedic Routine

Once you have identified your dosha, it's time to create a personalized Ayurvedic

routine. This routine will involve incorporating various health and beauty practices that balance your dosha and promote overall wellness.

Diet: Ayurveda emphasizes the importance of a balanced diet that suits your dosha.

Vata types may benefit from warm, grounding foods, while Pitta types may thrive on

cooling, hydrating foods. Kapha types may benefit from light, spicy foods that promote digestion. Including spices and herbs specific to your dosha can also enhance the

benefits.

Exercise: Engaging in regular physical activity is crucial for maintaining a healthy body and mind. However, the type and intensity of exercise may vary depending on your dosha.

Vata types may benefit from gentle exercises like yoga and walking, while Pitta types may enjoy more intense activities like swimming or biking. Kapha types may benefit from vigorous exercises that promote sweat and detoxification.

Skincare and Self-care: Ayurveda places great importance on skincare and self-care practices. Using natural ingredients and oils that suit your dosha can nourish and rejuvenate your skin. Incorporating self-care practices like oil massage, meditation, and breathing exercises can help balance your dosha and reduce stress.

By understanding your dosha and incorporating Ayurvedic practices into your daily

routine, you can enhance your health and beauty naturally.

Remember, Ayurveda is a journey of self-discovery and self-care, so embrace the process and enjoy the transformative benefits it brings to your life.

Ayurvedic Self-Care Practices for Busy Individuals

In today's fast-paced world, it can be challenging to find time to take care of ourselves. However, self-care is essential for maintaining optimal health and beauty.

Ayurveda, the ancient Indian system of medicine, offers a range of natural remedies and practices that can easily fit into a busy individual's lifestyle. By incorporating Ayurvedic self-care practices into your daily routine, you can enhance your overall well-being and radiate

natural beauty.

One of the key principles of Ayurveda is the concept of balance. It emphasizes the importance of maintaining a

harmonious equilibrium between mind, body, and spirit.

To achieve this, Ayurveda recommends following a daily routine, known as Dinacharya, which ncludes specific self-care practices tailored to your unique constitution or dosha.

To start your day on the right foot, Ayurveda suggests rising early, ideally before sunrise. This allows you to align with nature's rhythm and tap into its

healing energy.

Begin with tongue scraping, using a copper or stainless-steel tongue cleaner to remove toxins and promote oral hygiene.

Next, engage in self-massage, or Abhyanga, using warm herbal oils. This practice not only nourishes and hydrates the skin but also improves circulation and relaxes the mind. Focus on massaging the scalp, face, and body, paying attention to areas of tension or dryness.

Following your self-massage, practice Pranayama, or conscious breathing exercises. This helps

exercises. This helps to calm the mind, increase energy levels, and improve respiratory function.

Simple techniques like deep belly breathing or alternate nostril breathing can be done anywhere, even during a busy day at work.

Incorporating Ayurvedic dietary guidelines into your routine is also crucial for self-care. Aim to eat three balanced meals a day, emphasizing fresh, whole foods that are appropriate for your dosha. Avoid processed foods, excessive caffeine, and heavily spiced or fried foods, as they can disrupt your body's natural balance.

Finally, before bed, practice a calming bedtime routine to promote restful sleep. This may include gentle stretching, reading a book, or practicing meditation or mindfulness. Adequate sleep is vital for rejuvenation, and Ayurveda recommends aiming for seven to eight hours of uninterrupted rest each night.

By incorporating these Ayurvedic self-care practices into your busy schedule, you

can enhance your health and beauty naturally.

Remember, self-care is not selfish; it is an investment in your overall well-being. Take the time to prioritize yourself and experience the transformative power of Ayurveda in your daily life.

Ayurvedic Tips for Healthy Relationships

In today's fast-paced world,maintaining healthy relationships can be challenging. Stress, lack of time, and communication issues often take a toll on our relationships, leading to disharmony and discontent.

However, Ayurveda, the ancient Indian system of medicine and wellness, offers valuable insights and practices for nurturing healthy relationships

By incorporating Ayurvedic principles into our daily lives, we can enhance our relationships and foster a deeper sense of connection and love.

1. Understanding Doshas: According to Ayurveda, every individual has a unique mind-body constitution, known as dosha.

 Understanding your own dosha and that of your partner can provide valuable insights into your

personalities, preferences, and communication styles.

By understanding each other's doshas, you can adapt your interactions and create a more harmonious bond.

2. Practice Self-Care: Self-care is essential for maintaining healthy relationships. When you prioritize your own well-being, you become more

present, patient, and compassionate towards your loved ones. Incorporate Ayurvedic self-care practices such as Abhyanga (self-massage), meditation, and yoga into your routine to reduce stress and promote overall well-being.

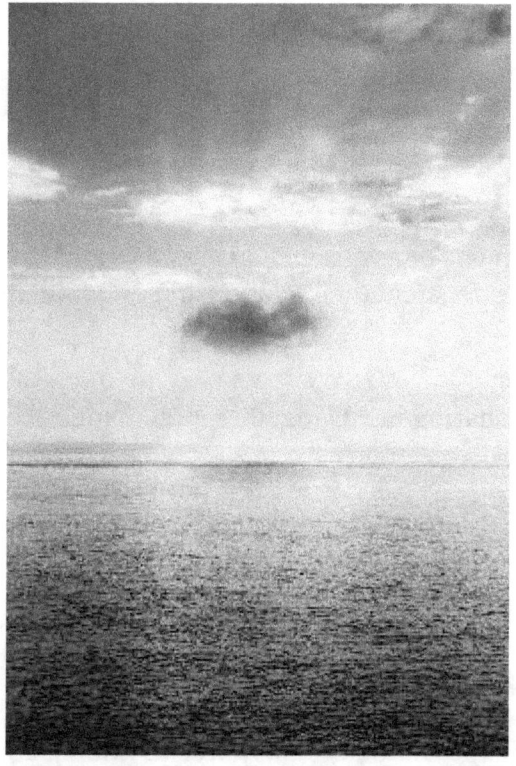

3. Nourish with Ayurvedic Diet: Ayurveda emphasizes the importance of food in maintaining balance and harmony. Cook and share meals together using fresh, seasonal ingredients.

Consider your doshas and incorporate Ayurvedic foods that support balance and vitality. For

example, Vata individuals can benefit from warm, grounding foods, while Pitta types can enjoy cooling and soothing foods.

4. Communication and Listening: Effective communication is thefoundation of any healthy relationship. Ayurveda emphasizes active listening and mindful speech. Practice active

listening by giving your full attention to your partner, without interrupting or

judging. Choose your words wisely, speaking with kindness and respect.

5. Rituals and Bonding Activities: Ayurveda encourages the practice of rituals and bonding activities to strengthen relationships.

Establish daily rituals such as sharing meals together, practicing gratitude, or taking

evening walks. These activities create a sense of togetherness and foster deeper connections.

6. Balance Work and Family Time: In today's busy world, finding a balance between work and family time is crucial. Ayurveda emphasizes the need for quality time with loved ones to

maintain healthy relationships. Prioritize spending time together, engaging in meaningful activities that bring joy and relaxation.

By incorporating these Ayurvedic tips into your life, you can enhance your relationships and create a harmonious and loving environment.

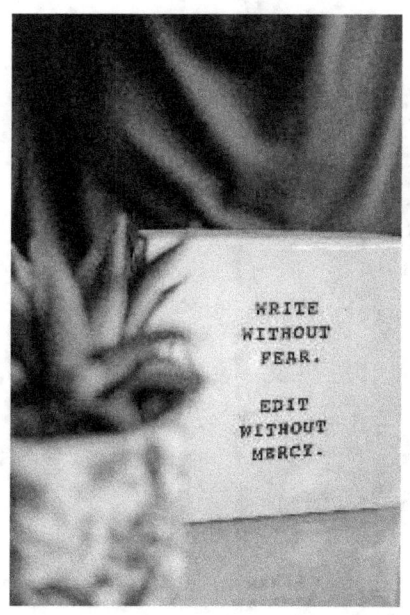

Remember, lasting relationships require ongoing effort, patience, and understanding. With Ayurveda as your guide, you can cultivate deep and meaningful connections that stand the test of time.

Ayurveda and Exercise

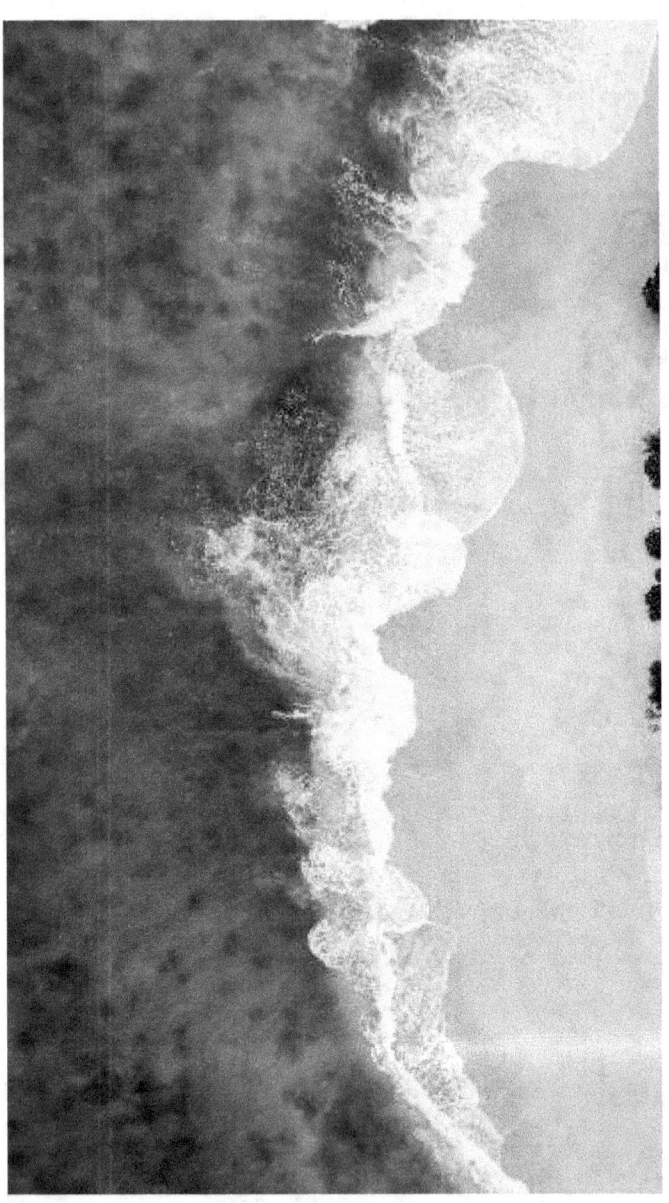

In the pursuit of good health and beauty, many of us turn to exercise as a means to achieve our goals. While modern forms of exercise have gained immense popularity,

Ayurveda offers a unique perspective on physical activity that goes beyond mere

physical fitness. Ayurvedic health and beauty practices emphasize the importance of balancing the mind, body, and spirit. Exercise, when approached with an Ayurvedic mindset, can become a powerful tool for achieving overall well-being.

According to Ayurveda, every individual possesses a unique constitution or "dosha" - Vata, Pitta, or Kapha. Understanding your dosha is essential when it comes to choosing the right exercise routine.

Vata types, who are prone to anxiety and restlessness, benefit from grounding exercises

such as yoga, tai chi, or walking in nature.

Pitta individuals, who tend to be competitive and fiery, should opt for activities that promote relaxation and cooling, such as swimming or gentle cycling.

Kapha individuals, who are naturally calm and easygoing but prone to lethargy, benefit from vigorous exercises like running, dancing, or high-intensity interval training.

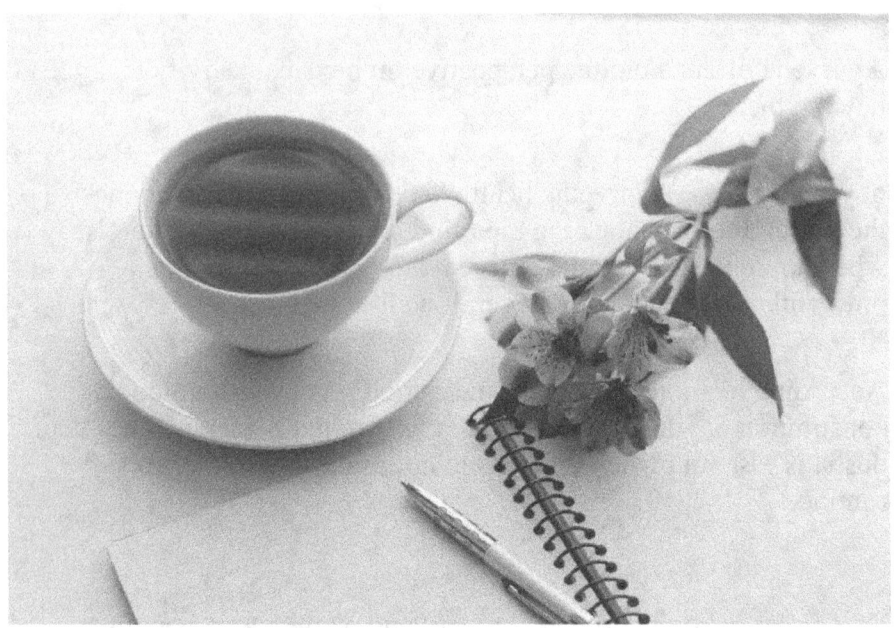

Ayurveda also emphasizes the importance of exercising at the right time of day. The ideal time for physical activity varies depending on an individual's dosha.

Vata types should exercise during the calm and stable period of the day, preferably in the morning. Pitta individuals should opt for cooler parts of the day, like early morning or evening,

To avoid overheating. Kapha types, on the other hand, benefit from exercising during the energetic and stimulating period of the day, which is typically in the late morning or early afternoon.

In addition to choosing the right exercise and timing, Ayurveda recommends incorporating other practices to enhance the benefits of physical activity. Pre-exercise rituals, such as

self-massage with warm oil, can help lubricate the joints and muscles, prevent injuries, and promote relaxation. Post-exercise routines, like gentle stretching and meditation, aid in

cooling down the body, calming the mind, and supporting recovery.

When approached with an Ayurvedic mindset, exercise becomes more than just a means to burn calories or build muscle. It becomes a holistic practice that aligns the mind, body, and

spirit, promoting overall health and beauty.

By understanding your dosha and choosing the right exercise routine and timing, you can optimize your physical activity to suit your unique constitution. Incorporating pre and post-exercise rituals further enhances the benefits,ensuring a well-rounded approach to fitness and well-being.

In conclusion, Ayurveda and exercise go hand in hand when it comes to enhancing health and beauty naturally. By embracing the principles of Ayurvedic health and beauty practices, you can transform your exercise routine into a personalized and holistic experience that

nurtures your entire being.

So, let Ayurveda be your guide on the path to vibrant health and radiant beauty through the power of exercise.

Ayurvedic Practices for Better Sleep

In today's fast-paced world, getting a good night's sleep has become increasingly elusive for many people

The constant stress, hectic schedules, and digital distractions often leave us tossing and turning in bed, unable to find the

restful sleep our bodies and minds

desperately need.

Thankfully, Ayurveda, the ancient Indian system of medicine and wellness, offers a holistic approach to achieving better sleep naturally.

By incorporating Ayurvedic practices into our daily routines, we can restore balance to our bodies and minds, promoting deep

and rejuvenating sleep.

One of the key principles of Ayurveda is understanding and honoring our unique mind-body constitution, or dosha. The three doshas – Vata, Pitta, and Kapha – influence our physical and mental characteristics, including our sleep patterns.

By identifying our dominant dosha, we can tailor our sleep rituals to address any imbalances and create an optimal sleep environment.

For Vata types, known for their active minds and restlessness, establishing a calming bedtime routine is essential. This may include gentle yoga stretches, warm baths infused with calming essential oils like lavender or chamomile, and sipping a warm cup of herbal tea before bed.

Creating a serene sleep environment with dim lighting, soothing music, and minimizing electronic devices in the bedroom can also promote better sleep.

Pitta types, on the other hand, benefit from cooling and relaxing practices to counter their fiery nature. Cooling breathing exercises such as Sheetali and Sheetkari can help calm the mind and body.

Additionally, using cooling essential oils like sandalwood or rose can be applied to the temples or added to a diffuser. Sleeping in a cool room with natural fibers like cotton or silk can also support better sleep for Pitta types.

Kapha types, known for their stability and tendency towards heaviness, may need to focus on energizing practices to counter daytime lethargy. Engaging in invigorating

exercises like brisk walks or yoga poses that stimulate circulation can be beneficial.

Aromatherapy with uplifting scents like citrus or eucalyptus can help awaken the

senses. Maintaining a well-ventilated sleep environment with natural light can also help Kapha types feel more refreshed upon awakening.

In addition to these dosha-specific practices, Ayurveda emphasizes the importance of maintaining a regular sleep-wake schedule, avoiding heavy meals close to bedtime, and cultivating a tranquil, clutter-free sleep environment.

By incorporating these Ayurvedic practices into our daily lives, we can promote restful sleep,

enhance our overall well-being, and awaken each morning feeling rejuvenated and ready to take on the day.

Remember, the practices mentioned here are general recommendations, and it's always best to consult with an Ayurvedic practitioner to understand your unique constitution and receive personalized guidance.

By embracing the wisdom of Ayurveda, we can embark on a journey towards better sleep and a healthier, more balanced life.

Recommended Books on Ayurveda

Ayurveda, offers a holistic approach to achieving optimal health and beauty

naturally. If you are interested in delving deeper in to the principles and practices of Ayurveda, here are some highly

recommended books that will provide you with valuable insights and guidance.

1. "The Complete Book of Ayurvedic Home Remedies" by Dr. Vasant Lad
Considered a classic in the field, this book is

an excellent resource for anyone seeking self-

care solutions using Ayurvedic principles. Dr. Vasant Lad, one of the foremost Ayurvedic practitioners in the West, provides easy-to-

understand explanations of Ayurvedic concepts and offers practical remedies for common ailments and imbalances.

2. "Ayurveda: The Science of Self- Healing" by Dr. Vasant Lad
Another gem by Dr. Vasant Lad, this book explores the fundamental principles of Ayurveda and how they can be applied to

restore and maintain good health. It covers various aspects, including diet, lifestyle,

herbal remedies, and detoxification

techniques, making it an essential guide for beginners and those seeking to

deepen their understanding.

3. "The Ayurveda Bible" by Anne McIntyre Anne McIntyre, a renowned Ayurvedic practitioner and herbalist, presents acomprehensive guide to Ayurvedic

principles, practices, and remedies in this well-organized book.

It covers a wide range of topics, including diet, lifestyle, yoga, meditation, beauty treatments, and herbal medicine, making

it a valuable resource for those looking to incorporate Ayurveda into their daily lives.

4. "The Everyday Cookbook" by Kate O'Donnell
For those interested in Ayurveda's culinary traditions, this cookbook by

Kate O'Donnell is a must-have. It offers a diverse collection of vegetarian recipes that are not only delicious but also tailored to balance the doshas in. the body.

With easy-to-follow instructions and helpful tips, this book allows you to explore the healing power of Ayurvedic cooking in your own kitchen.

These recommended books on Ayurveda provide a comprehensive

understanding of this ancient system of medicine and its application in

promoting health and beauty naturally.

Whether you are new to Ayurveda or have some prior knowledge, these

resources will empower you to

incorporate Ayurvedic principles into your daily routines and enhance your overall well-being.

Through her own experiences, she offers wisdom on balancing the body, mind, and spirit, and provides practical guidance on diet, lifestyle, and self-care practices. This book is especially beneficial for those seeking a deeper connection with Ayurveda's spiritual aspects. lifestyle, and self-care practices.

In conclusion, the internet is a treasure trove of information when it comes to Ayurveda.

Whether you prefer reading articles, watching videos, engaging in discussions, or taking online courses, there are countless resources available to enhance your knowledge of Ayurvedic health and beauty practices.

Embrace the digital era and explore these online resources to embark on a journey towards natural wellness and timeless beauty.

Online Resources for Ayurvedic Information

In this digital age, the internet has become an invaluable tool for accessing

information on various topics. Ayurveda, the ancient Indian system of medicine and well-being, is no exception.

If you are interested in learning more about Ayurvedic health and beauty practices, there are numerous online resources available to guide you on your journey towards natural wellness. Websites dedicated to Ayurveda provide a wealth of information on various topics, including understanding Ayurvedic principles, discovering individual body types or doshas, and learning about specific Ayurvedic treatments and techniques.

One such website is "Ayurveda for All," which offers a comprehensive guide to Ayurvedic concepts and practices. It covers everything from basic principles to Ayurvedic dietary recommendations and herbal remedies.

For those who prefer video content, YouTube has a vast collection of Ayurveda-related channels that offer informative videos on a wide range of topics. Channels like "Ayurvedic Healing" and "The Ayurveda Experience" provide tutorials, interviews with experts, and practical tips for incorporating Ayurveda into your daily life.

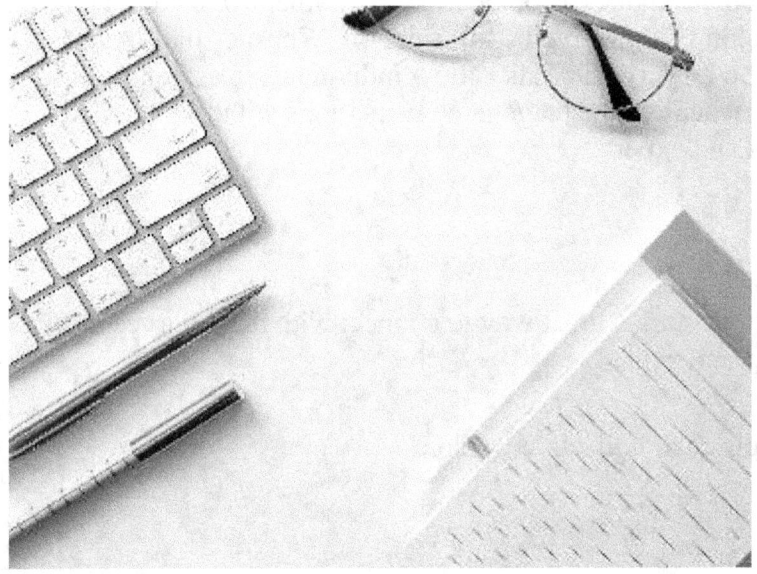

These videos are a great way to visually understand Ayurvedic practices and learn from experienced practitioners.

Social media platforms like Instagram and Facebook also serve as valuable resources for Ayurvedic information. Many Ayurvedic practitioners and wellness influencers share their knowledge and experiences through posts and live videos. Following these accounts can provide you with daily inspiration, tips, and insights into Ayurvedic health and beauty practices.

Online forums and discussion boards are another avenue to explore when searching for Ayurvedic information. Websites like "Ayurveda Forums" and "Ayurvedic Talk" allow individuals to ask questions, share experiences, and engage in conversations with like-minded individuals and experts.

These platforms are a great way to connect with the Ayurvedic community and gain

insights from their collective wisdom.

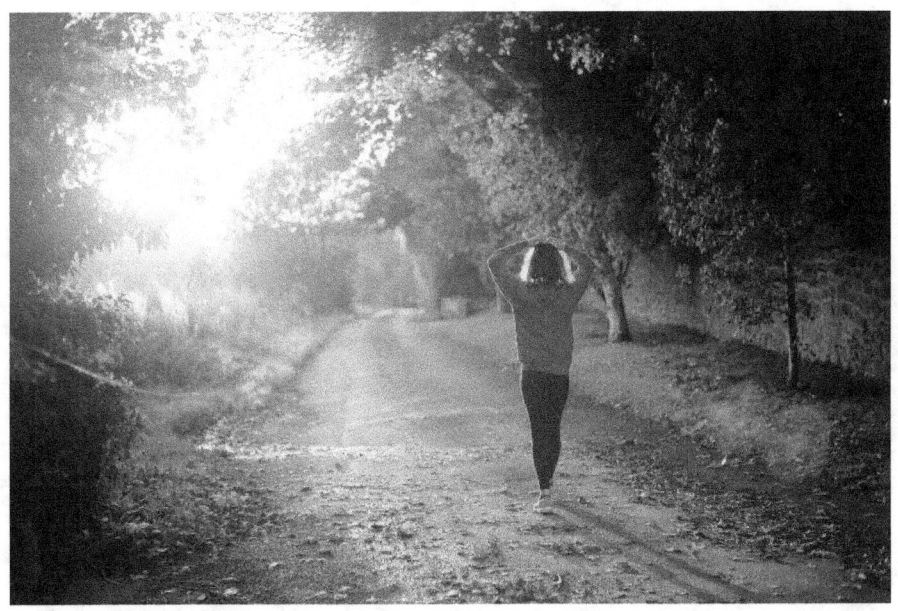

Lastly, online courses and webinars offer a more structured approach to learning Ayurveda.

Websites like "Ayurveda Institute" and "Ayurveda College" provide comprehensive courses

taught by experienced Ayurvedic practitioners. These courses cover a wide range of topics, from Ayurvedic nutrition to herbal medicine, and offer a more in-depth understanding of the principles and practices of Ayurveda.

In conclusion, the internet is a treasure trove of information when it comes to Ayurveda.

Whether you prefer reading articles, watching videos, engaging in discussions, or taking online courses, there are countless resources available to enhance your knowledge of Ayurvedic health and beauty practices.

Embrace the digital era and explore these online resources to embark on a journey towards natural wellness and timeless beauty.

Ayurvedic Practitioners and Retreats

In this chapter, we will explore the role of Ayurvedic practitioners and the benefits of Ayurvedic retreats. Ayurveda, an ancient Indian system of medicine, offers a holistic approach to health and beauty. By understanding the principles of Ayurveda, you can

enhance your well-being naturally.

Ayurvedic Practitioners:

Ayurvedic practitioners play a vital role in guiding individuals towards optimal health. These professionals have undergone extensive training and possess in-depth knowledge of

Ayurvedic principles and practices. They offer personalized consultations, where they assess your unique constitution (dosha) and provide tailored recommendations for diet, lifestyle, and herbal remedies.

Whether you are seeking relief from a specific ailment or simply aiming to improve your overall health, an Ayurvedic practitioner can assist you on your wellness journey.

With the help of experienced practitioners, you can gain deeper insights into your own well-being and make positive changes in your life.

Benefits of Ayurvedic Retreats:
Ayurvedic retreats provide an immersive experience where you can fully immerse yourself in the healing aspects of Ayurveda. These retreats offer a variety of activities such as yoga, meditation, and self-awareness.

Ayurvedic retreats focus on treating the mind, body, and spirit as a whole. Through various therapies and practices, these retreats aim to restore balance and harmony within you.Here are some notable benefits of attending an Ayurvedic retreat:

Ayurvedic retreats provide an immersive experience where you can fully immerse yourself in the healing aspects of Ayurveda.

Ayurvedic retreats provide an immersive experience where you can fully immerse yourself in the healing aspects of Ayurveda. These retreats offer a variety of activities such as yoga, meditation, and self-awareness.

1. Detoxification: Ayurvedic retreats often include detoxification programs to eliminate toxins from the body. These programs may

involve specific dietary regimes, herbaltreatments, and rejuvenating therapies.

2. Stress Reduction: Ayurvedic retreats provide a tranquil environment away from the hustle and bustle of everyday life. By engaging in relaxation techniques like meditation and Ayurvedic massages, you can release stress and find inner peace.

3. Education and Empowerment: Ayurvedic retreats offer educational workshops and seminars where you can learn about Ayurvedic principles and practices. This knowledge empowers you to make informed choices about your health and beauty routines even after the retreat ends.

health and beauty routines even after the retreat ends.

4. Self-Discovery and Personal Growth: Ayurvedic retreats encourage self-reflection and self-awareness.

Through introspection and guidance from Ayurvedic retreats offer educational workshops and seminars where you can learn about Ayurvedic principles and practices. Ayurvedic retreats offer educational workshops and seminars where you can learn about Ayurvedic principles and practices.

Attending an Ayurvedic retreat allows you to immerse yourself in the wisdom of Ayurveda, rejuvenate your body and mind, and gain valuable knowledge toincorporate Ayurvedic practices into your daily life.

Whether you choose to consult with an Ayurvedic practitioner or embark on an Ayurvedic retreat, these experiences offer a holistic approach to health and beauty.

By embracing Ayurveda, you can enhance your well-being naturally and achieve a balanced and harmonious life.

Ayurveda and Certification Programs

In recent years, there has been a growing interest in Ayurveda, the ancient Indian system of medicine that focuses on achieving balance and harmony in the body, mind, and spirit.

As more people recognize the benefits of Ayurvedic health and beauty practices, the demand for certified Ayurvedic practitioners has also increased.

This chapter aims to provide an overview of Ayurveda certification programs and their significance in the field.

spirit. As more people recognize the benefits of Ayurvedic health and beauty practices, the demand for certified Ayurvedic practitioners has also increased. This chapter aims to provide an overview of Ayurveda certification programs and their significance in the field.

Ayurveda certification programs offer individuals the

opportunity to deepen their knowledge and understanding of this holistic approach to health and beauty. These programs are designed to equip students with the skills and expertise required to practice Ayurveda professionally. Whether you aspire to become

an Ayurvedic consultant, therapist, or educator, obtaining certification is an important step towards establishing yourself in the field.

One of the key advantages of enrolling in an Ayurveda certification program is that it provides a structured and comprehensive curriculum.

These programs cover a wide range of topics, including the principles of Ayurveda, anatomy and physiology, herbal medicine, diet and nutrition, yoga and meditation, and Ayurvedic therapies.

By studying these subjects, students gain a deep understanding of Ayurveda's core principles and learn how to apply them in real-life situations.

Moreover, Ayurveda certification programs often involve practical training and hands-on experience. Students have the opportunity to work with experienced Ayurvedic practitioners and learn directly from them. This practical component allows students to refine their skills and gain confidence in applying Ayurvedic principles to promote health and beauty.

Furthermore, obtaining certification demonstrates a commitment to professionalism and

ethics in the practice of Ayurveda. Certified Ayurvedic practitioners are recognized for their expertise and adherence to high standards of care. This recognition not only

enhances their credibility but also instills trust and confidence in clients seeking Ayurvedic services.

It is important to note that certification requirements may vary depending on the

country or region. Some programs may offer basic certifications, while others provide advanced levels of training.

Before enrolling in a program, it is advisable to research and choose one that aligns with your goals and aspirations.

In conclusion, Ayurveda certification programs play a vital role in the field of Ayurvedic health and beauty practices.

They provide individuals with the knowledge, skills, and practical experience necessary to practice

Ayurveda professionally. By obtaining certification, practitioners demonstrate their commitment to professionalism, ethics, and the well-being of their

clients.

Whether you are considering a career in Ayurveda or simply want to deepen your understanding of this ancient system, enrolling in a certification program can be a transformative experience.

Continuing Your Ayurvedic Journey

Congratulations on taking the first step towards enhancing your health and

beauty naturally with Ayurveda!

Now that you have gained an understanding of the basic principles and practices of this ancient healing system, it's time to embark on a journey that will transform your life.

Ayurveda is a holistic approach to health and beauty that focuses on balancing the mind, body, and spirit. It emphasizes the importance of harmony between these elements to achieve overal

well-being. By following Ayurvedic practices, you can not only improve your physical health but also enhance your natural beauty.

As you continue your Ayurvedic journey, it is crucial to remember that consistency is key. Incorporating Ayurvedic practices into your daily routine will yield the best results.

Start by identifying your dosha, or mind-body type, to customize your health and beauty regimen accordingly.

For those with a Vata dosha, which is characterized by qualities of air and space, focus on grounding and nourishing practices. Incorporate warm, cooked foods into your diet and engage in activities that promote stability and relaxation, such as yoga and meditation. Use oils like sesame or almond for self-massage to moisturize and calm your skin.

Pitta dosha individuals, who have qualities of fire and water, should prioritize cooling and calming practices. Opt for a diet rich in fresh fruits and vegetables, and avoid spicy or oily

foods. Engage in activities that promote balance and flexibility, such as swimming or walking in nature. Use cooling oils like coconut or rose for your skincare routine.

Kapha dosha individuals, characterized by earth and water qualities, should

focus on invigorating and energizing practices. Include spices and light, warming foods in your diet, and

engage in vigorous activities like dancing or aerobics. Use light, non-greasy oils like jojoba or grapeseed for your skincare routine.

In addition to these personalized practices, there are several Ayurvedic rituals that benefit everyone.

Daily self- care rituals, known as Dinacharya, include tongue scraping, oil pulling, and dry brushing, which help remove toxins and promote overall well-being.

Furthermore, Ayurveda encourages the use of natural ingredients for beauty care. Explore the benefits of herbs like turmeric, neem, and aloe vera for your skincare routine.

Experiment with homemade face masks,
hair oils, and body scrubs using these natural

ingredients to enhance your beauty naturally.

Remember, Ayurveda is not a quick fix but a lifestyle. Be patient and consistent in your Ayurvedic practices, and you will gradually

witness the transformative effects on your health and beauty. Embrace this holistic approach, and let Ayurveda guide you towards a healthier and more beautiful you.

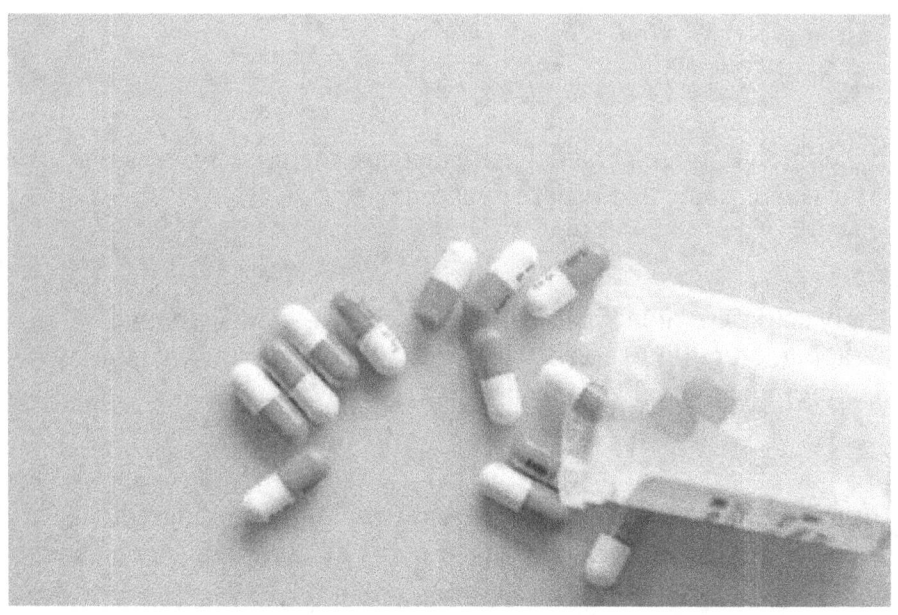

Continue your Ayurvedic journey with an open mind and a willingness to explore

new practices. Your commitment to this ancient healing system will reward you with long-lasting health and radiant

beauty. Enjoy the process, and may your Ayurvedic journey be a fulfilling and

enriching one.

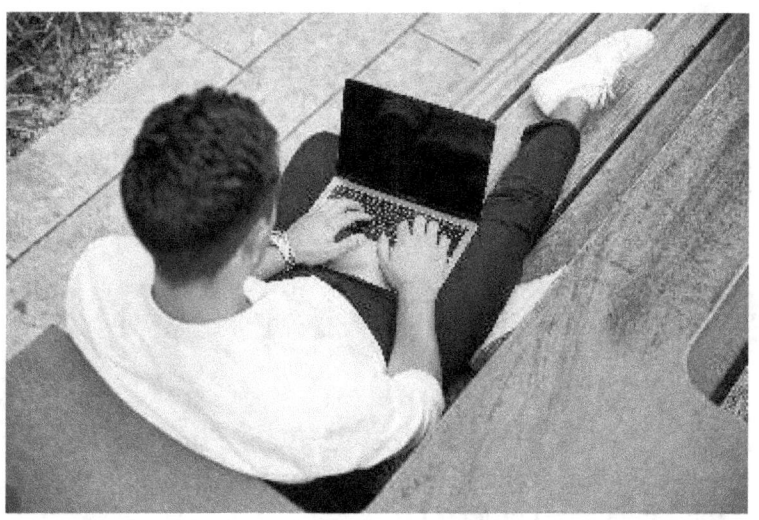

Recap of Ayurvedic Principles and Practices

Welcome back to "Ayurveda Simplified."

In this chapter, we will take a moment to recap the fundamental principles and practices of Ayurveda, the ancient Indian system of medicine and wellness.

Whether you are new to Ayurveda or seeking a refresher, this recap will serve as a valuable reference for your journey towards holistic well-being.

Ayurveda, meaning "Science of Life," is based on the belief that health is a harmonious balance between the mind, body, and spirit. It emphasizes prevention and self-care, aiming to address the root causes of imbalances rather than merely treating symptoms. By

understanding and applying Ayurvedic principles, you can enhance your health and beauty naturally.

One of the key principles of Ayurveda is the concept of doshas, which are the three

fundamental energies that govern our bodies: Vata, Pitta, and Kapha. Each person has a unique combination of these doshas, and maintaining their balance is crucial for

optimal health. Ayurvedic practices, such as diet, lifestyle modifications, and herbal remedies, are tailored to individual doshic imbalances.

Ayurveda also promotes the importance of daily routines, or dinacharya, to establish

harmony and balance in our lives. This includes practices such as tongue scraping, oil

pulling, self-massage (abhyanga), and meditation. These rituals not only nurture the body but also calm the mind and awaken the spirit, leading to a more vibrant and joyful existence.

When it comes to Ayurvedic health and beauty practices, understanding your

skin type and incorporating suitable

skincare routines is essential.

Ayurveda recognizes that external beauty

is a reflection of internal health. Thus, it emphasizes nourishing the skin with

natural ingredients, such as herbs, oils, and minerals, to maintain a radiant

complexion.

Ayurveda also offers a wide range of herbal remedies and natural ingredients that can be used for various beauty treatments. From turmeric for brightening the skin to amla for promoting hair growth, Ayurvedic herbs have been used for centuries to enhance beauty naturally. By incorporating these ingredients into your skincare and haircare routines, you can tap into the power of nature for a naturally radiant appearance.

Furthermore, Ayurveda recognizes the mind-body connection and the impact of stress on overall well-being. Through practices such as meditation, yoga, and pranayama

(breathing exercises), Ayurveda helps to reduce stress, promote relaxation, and

cultivate a sense of inner peace. By incorporating these practices into your daily life, you can enhance both your physical and mental well-being, which ultimately reflects in your outer beauty.

In conclusion, embracing Ayurveda for enhanced health and beauty is a holistic

approach that encompasses various aspects of our lives – from diet and self-care rituals to herbal remedies and stress management techniques.

By incorporating Ayurvedic practices into your daily routine, you can nurture your body, mind, and spirit, and achieve a natural and radiant beauty that shines from within.

Your Ayurvedic Journey Begins Now!

patterns. Once you have identified your dosha(s), you can tailor your health and beauty practices accordingly.

Ayurveda offers a plethora of natural remedies and practices to promote well-being. From dietaryrecommendations to herbal therapies, from meditation to yoga, Ayurveda

encompasses a wide range of techniques to restore balance and vitality.

One of the key aspects of Ayurveda is nourishing your body from the inside out. We have explored the importance of a sattvic diet – a diet that promotes purity, clarity, and vitality and the six tastes and how to incorporate them into your meals to maintain balance.

. We also discussed the benefits of Ayurvedic herbs and spices and how they can be

Additionally, Ayurveda emphasizes the importance of self-care rituals and daily routines, known as dinacharya. We will guide you through establishing a personalized morning and evening routine that aligns with your dosha constitution.

From oil pulling to tongue scraping, from Abhyanga (self-massage) to Nasya (nasal cleansing), you will discover simple yet powerful practices to enhance your well- being.

Hopefully, you will have gained a solid foundation in Ayurvedic health and beauty practices

and be equipped with the knowledge and tools to embark on your Ayurvedic journey,

promoting balance, vitality, and radiance in your life.
]
Get ready to embrace the wisdom of Ayurveda and unlock the secrets to natural health and beauty!